ARE WE READY TO LIVE 150 YEARS?

EXPLORING THE FUTURE OF LONGEVITY

DAVID SANDUA

Are we ready to live 150 years?. Exploring the future of longevity.
© David Sandua 2024. All rights reserved.
Electronic and paperback edition.

"By 2050, the idea of living to 150 years will be common, thanks to advances in biotechnology and nanotechnology."

Peter Diamandis (Businessman and futurist)

INDEX

I. INTRODUCTION ... 10
- OVERVIEW OF LONGEVITY TRENDS ... 11
- IMPORTANCE OF THE TOPIC ... 14
- OBJECTIVES OF THE ESSAY ... 15

II. HISTORICAL PERSPECTIVES ON LONGEVITY ... 18
- EVOLUTION OF LIFE EXPECTANCY ... 20
- KEY MILESTONES IN AGING RESEARCH ... 22
- CULTURAL ATTITUDES TOWARDS AGING ... 24

III. SCIENTIFIC FOUNDATIONS OF AGING ... 27
- BIOLOGICAL MECHANISMS OF AGING ... 29
- THEORIES OF AGING ... 30
- RECENT DISCOVERIES IN GERONTOLOGY ... 32

IV. TECHNOLOGICAL INNOVATIONS IN LONGEVITY ... 35
- ADVANCES IN BIOTECHNOLOGY ... 37
- ROLE OF ARTIFICIAL INTELLIGENCE ... 39
- IMPACT OF WEARABLE HEALTH TECHNOLOGY ... 41

V. REGENERATIVE MEDICINE ... 44
- STEM CELL RESEARCH ... 46
- TISSUE ENGINEERING ... 47
- ORGAN REGENERATION TECHNIQUES ... 49

VI. GENETIC EDITING AND LONGEVITY ... 52
- CRISPR AND ITS IMPLICATIONS ... 54
- ETHICAL CONSIDERATIONS OF GENETIC MODIFICATION ... 55
- POTENTIAL FOR DISEASE PREVENTION ... 57

VII. NUTRITIONAL SCIENCE AND LONGEVITY ... 60
- ROLE OF DIET IN AGING ... 62
- CALORIC RESTRICTION AND ITS EFFECTS ... 63
- SUPPLEMENTS AND LONGEVITY ... 66

VIII. MENTAL HEALTH AND LONGEVITY ... 68
- PSYCHOLOGICAL WELL-BEING IN OLD AGE ... 69
- COGNITIVE DECLINE AND PREVENTION ... 71
- SOCIAL CONNECTIONS AND LONGEVITY ... 73

IX. ECONOMIC IMPLICATIONS OF EXTENDED LIFESPAN ... 76
- IMPACT ON HEALTHCARE SYSTEMS ... 78
- WORKFORCE DYNAMICS AND RETIREMENT ... 80
- ECONOMIC OPPORTUNITIES IN LONGEVITY INDUSTRIES ... 82

X. ETHICAL DILEMMAS OF LONGEVITY ... 85
- EQUITY IN ACCESS TO LONGEVITY TECHNOLOGIES ... 87
- MORAL IMPLICATIONS OF LIFE EXTENSION ... 89
- THE VALUE OF LIFE AND DEATH ... 91

XI. SOCIAL DYNAMICS OF AN AGING POPULATION ... 94
- CHANGING FAMILY STRUCTURES ... 96
- INTERGENERATIONAL RELATIONSHIPS ... 98
- COMMUNITY SUPPORT SYSTEMS ... 100

XII. CULTURAL PERSPECTIVES ON AGING 102
Variations in Attitudes Across Cultures 104
Rituals and Traditions Surrounding Aging 106
Global Perspectives on Longevity 107

XIII. POLICY CONSIDERATIONS FOR LONGEVITY 110
Government Regulations on Biotechnology 112
Public Health Initiatives 114
Funding for Aging Research 116

XIV. ENVIRONMENTAL SUSTAINABILITY AND LONGEVITY 119
Resource Management for an Aging Population 121
Impact of Longevity on Climate Change 122
Sustainable Practices for Long Life 125

XV. QUALITY OF LIFE IN OLD AGE 127
Defining Quality of Life 129
Health span vs. Lifespan 131
Enhancing Life Satisfaction 133

XVI. THE ROLE OF TECHNOLOGY IN ELDER CARE 135
Telehealth and Remote Monitoring 136
Robotics in Assisted Living 138
Smart Homes for Seniors 140

XVII. THE FUTURE OF WORK IN AN AGING SOCIETY 143
Lifelong Learning and Employment 145
Age Diversity in the Workplace 147
Adapting Work Environments for Older Adults 149

XVIII. LONGEVITY AND GLOBAL HEALTH 151
Health Disparities and Longevity 152
Global Aging Trends 155
International Collaboration in Aging Research 157

XIX. PSYCHOLOGICAL ADAPTATION TO LONGEVITY 160
Coping with Extended Lifespan 161
Identity and Self-Perception in Old Age 163
Resilience and Aging 165

XX. THE ROLE OF COMMUNITY IN LONGEVITY 168
Social Engagement and Longevity 170
Community Resources for Seniors 171
Volunteerism and Its Benefits 174

XXI. INNOVATIONS IN PALLIATIVE CARE 176
Importance of End-of-Life Care 178
Advances in Pain Management 180
Holistic Approaches to Palliative Care 182

XXII. THE IMPACT OF LONGEVITY ON EDUCATION 185
Lifelong Learning Opportunities 186
Educational Programs for Older Adults 188
Intergenerational Learning 191

XXIII. FUTURE RESEARCH DIRECTIONS IN LONGEVITY 193
Emerging Fields of Study 195
Interdisciplinary Approaches 197
Funding and Support for Research 198

XXIV. CASE STUDIES OF LONGEVITY 201
Blue Zones and Their Secrets 203
Successful Aging Models 205
Lessons from Centenarians 207

XXV. PUBLIC PERCEPTION OF LONGEVITY 210
Media Representation of Aging 211
Public Awareness Campaigns 213
Attitudes Toward Longevity Technologies 215

XXVI. CONCLUSION 218
Summary of Key Findings 219
Implications for Society 221
Future Outlook on Longevity 223
Final Thoughts on Readiness for Extended Life 225

REFERENCES 227

I. INTRODUCTION

In recent years, discussions surrounding human longevity have intensified, driven by rapid advancements in science and technology. Emerging innovations in fields such as biotechnology, regenerative medicine, and genetic editing have ignited a conversation about the feasibility of extending human life significantly—possibly even reaching 150 years. As researchers unveil biological mechanisms associated with aging, such as senescence, telomere shortening, and mitochondrial dysfunction, the quest for prolonged life becomes more grounded in scientific inquiry. The promise of these advancements raises critical questions about our readiness to embrace lives that extend well beyond current expectations. A profound statement in this discourse suggests, The human lifespan is not fixed, and it has increased significantly over the past century. This assertion highlights our potential to utilize contemporary breakthroughs in health sciences to continue redefining the boundaries of human lifespan. The exploration of these themes carries implications not just for individual longevity but also for the entire socioeconomic landscape. Investing in the future of longevity presents significant ethical, economic, and social challenges that society must confront. As life expectancy increases, we must consider the impact on family structures, workforce dynamics, and healthcare systems. Potential implications could include increased intergenerational relationships, shifting economic responsibilities, and new cultural paradigms surrounding aging. If individuals live longer, the expectations for traditional milestones such as marriage, careers, and retirement may shift dramatically, leading to a re-evaluation of societal norms. The associated healthcare costs for an aging population could strain existing systems, necessitating innovative frameworks for elderly care and health maintenance. The integration of deep generative reinforcement learning and other advanced methodologies highlighted in various scientific studies may play a crucial role in developing sustainable health interventions. As we begin to formulate policies and social structures around longer lives, the importance of deliberate planning cannot be overstated. In contemplating the prospect of living longer, we must also address the implications for quality of life and human experience. While science pushes the boundaries of lifespan, the ultimate goal must remain focused on preserving vitality and well-being throughout extended years. Addressing factors that contribute to healthy aging, such as diet, mental health, and physical activity, will be essential in harnessing the benefits of longer lifespans. This holistic approach to health can mitigate risks associated with chronic conditions that often accompany aging, ensuring that extended years do not equate to prolonged suffering. Research into restoring biological function—evident from the exploration of aging clocks and multi-omics assessments—offers promising avenues for enhancing the quality of life as we age. As we stand on the precipice of potentially transformative changes in human longevity, it is imperative to consider not just how long we live, but how well we live.

Overview of Longevity Trends

Technological advancements have dramatically reshaped our understanding of health and longevity, offering unprecedented avenues for life extension. Innovations in biotechnology, such as gene editing and regenerative medicine, are paving the way for not only longevity but also improvements in the quality of life as individuals age. Researchers are increasingly focused on discoveries that target the fundamental biological processes responsible for aging, including cellular senescence and mitochondrial dysfunction. Insights gathered from interdisciplinary fields are forming the basis for new interventions aimed at delaying the onset of age-related diseases. As our grasp of these biological mechanisms deepens, the notion of living well into our 150s becomes less fantastical and more feasible. This trend is underscored by the observation that many individuals today possess a biologically younger profile compared to their chronological age, emphasizing that advancing age may not equate to declining vitality. illustrates these pathways clearly, linking deep learning methodologies with emerging fields in health research. Cultural perceptions significantly influence how societies respond to advancements in longevity science, impacting policy, healthcare systems, and individual aspirations. Diverse cultural attitudes towards aging determine the acceptance and integration of life-extending technologies into everyday life. Cultures that view aging as a natural process may exhibit resistance to interventions that challenge traditional beliefs regarding the life course. Conversely, societies embracing technological progress often celebrate the potential for enhanced longevity, fueling investment in related scientific research. As a result, contrasting perspectives may lead to significant disparities in health outcomes and access to innovations. An informed understanding of these cultural dynamics is crucial as we navigate the promises and challenges of longevity research. As we reflect on these trends, one cannot ignore the startling reality that, according to statistics, humans now have shorter attention spans than goldfish, exacerbated by lifestyle changes, which could hinder our ability to focus on sustaining longevity initiatives in the long term. The implications of extended lifespans extend beyond individual experiences, rippling through familial, social, and economic structures. Family dynamics are likely to shift as multiple generations coexist for longer periods, necessitating adjustments in caregiving and support systems. The workplace will also evolve, potentially leading to changes in retirement age, employment policies, and even the introduction of new professions to address the needs of an aging population. These prospects are accompanied by pressing ethical and social dilemmas. The societal focus must blend the pursuit of longevity with considerations of quality of life, equitable access to advancements, and the environmental impacts of a growing population. Emphasizing sustainable practices will be crucial in ensuring that the benefits of longevity are not overshadowed by increased resource consumption. The framework presented in reinforces this by visualizing ecological and systemic complexities that arise as we reconsider our approach to aging and health in an evolving world.

Year	Global Life Expectancy (Years)	Countries Over 80 Years (Count)	Notable Increases (%)
2020	72.6	40	1.2
2021	73.2	42	0.8
2022	73.4	45	0.3
2023	73.5	46	0.1
2024	74	48	0.7

Longevity Trends Overview

Importance of the Topic

Advancements in longevity research have opened new avenues for understanding the biological mechanisms underlying aging, thus reshaping societal perceptions of life expectancy. As scientists explore intricate relationships between genomic integrity, cellular senescence, and environmental factors, frameworks for comprehensive health strategies are becoming apparent. The illustration of biological aging processes, as detailed in, emphasizes critical interactions that contribute to longevity, such as cellular communication and nutrient regulation. This research not only identifies potential interventions but also underlines the necessity of a systems approach to health that transcends simplistic views of aging. As we navigate these advancements, it becomes paramount to educate communities about the implications of longevity, ensuring they are equipped to adapt to changing health paradigms and lifestyle adjustments. Living longer must not simply extend lifespan; it should enhance the quality of life, allowing individuals to remain active and engaged, addressing the fundamental challenge of achieving a higher life quality in advanced age. Addressing the ethical dimensions of prolonged life and its societal impacts is vital for shaping sustainable policies that govern future healthcare practices. These considerations urge us to interrogate our current frameworks and practices, asking whether they accommodate a world where individuals may live into their 150s. The complexities of this topic are highlighted by varying cultural responses to increased longevity, as communities around the globe react differently to the profound implications of these advancements. By assessing various attitudes toward aging, we can glean critical insights into developing inclusive policies that reflect diverse perspectives. The diagrammatic representation of the biological bases of aging provided in illustrates multiple determinants influencing longevity, enabling policymakers to tailor health initiatives that resonate with their local contexts. Fostering dialogue around these ethical challenges is essential, as it ensures that advancements are directed toward equitable health solutions that cater to the needs of all demographics. The integration of deep learning and artificial intelligence in health analysis showcases the transformative potential of technology in shaping our understanding of aging. By leveraging vast amounts of biological data as depicted in, researchers can uncover patterns that inform interventions and therapies aimed at mitigating age-related decline. This intersection of technology and health is not merely an academic exercise; it has profound implications for how we approach healthcare delivery in an aging society. As noted in, living longer creates opportunities for individuals to engage meaningfully in life, yet this necessitates a reevaluation of our social and economic systems. The promise of longevity must be accompanied by a commitment to innovate and adapt our infrastructures accordingly, ensuring that health advancements translate into accessible care for all. By embracing a comprehensive approach that melds technology, education, and community involvement, we can not only prepare for the challenges of aging societies but also celebrate the potential for enriched lives enhanced by scientific progress.

Objectives of the Essay

The exploration of longevity and the feasibility of extending human life to 150 years presents a multifaceted discourse that requires clarification of essential objectives. One goal of this essay is to analyze the scientific and technological advancements that underlie the increasing possibility of significant life extension. These advancements include breakthroughs in biotechnology, regenerative medicine, and genetic editing, each acting as a catalyst for rethinking health, aging, and disease management. By systematically evaluating these innovations, the essay illuminates how our understanding of aging and biological processes is evolving, leading to promising therapies that could one day revolutionize how we perceive the human lifespan. In doing so, it aims to create a clear narrative that captures the intersection of science and societal implications, thus providing critical insights into the plausibility of achieving a lifespan of 150 years, reinforcing a view that aligns with the overarching theme: The ultimate goal of longevity research is to understand the underlying biological mechanisms that contribute to aging and age-related diseases. Another objective of this examination is to scrutinize the ethical, economic, and social challenges accompanying the pursuit of extended lifespans. The prospect of living for 150 years elicits numerous concerns ranging from healthcare accessibility to eco-sustainability. The essay seeks to address how such unprecedented longevity might reshape family dynamics, labor markets, and social structures, revealing potential risks and rewards inherent in these transformations. As life expectancy potentially extends, societal expectations will need to adapt, leading to critical discussions surrounding the quality of life in older age. On this note, the investigation aims to provide a comprehensive understanding of how equitable access to life-extending advancements can be ensured in order to prevent disparities that such breakthroughs may inadvertently create. This discourse not only centers on scientific possibilities but also emphasizes the necessary ethical frameworks that must evolve in tandem with these advancements to ensure a meaningful extension of life. An exploration of differing cultural perspectives on aging and longevity is crucial in contextualizing societal reactions to the potential of living up to 150 years. Variations in societal attitudes toward aging can significantly influence the acceptance and implementation of biotechnologies aimed at extending life. This essay will delve into how different cultures perceive aging as a natural progression versus a condition to be modified or transcended. By analyzing these differing viewpoints, the discussion seeks to determine how cultural narratives can shape public perceptions and policy decisions related to longevity. Each culture's unique relationship with aging presents opportunities for learning and collaboration, potentially leading to a more inclusive approach to longevity research and its applications. The essay aims to foster a multidimensional understanding of longevity that respects cultural variations while advancing the dialogue about how humanity prepares for an increasingly prolonged existence.

II. HISTORICAL PERSPECTIVES ON LONGEVITY

The pursuit of longevity has captivated societies throughout history, deeply intertwined with cultural beliefs and practices. Ancient civilizations, such as the Greeks and Egyptians, often viewed aging and death through a spiritual lens, attributing longevity to divine favor or the intervention of gods. This perspective fostered a variety of rituals and lifestyle adjustments aimed at appeasing deities and nurturing vitality. In more recent history, the rise of empirical science has shifted the focus from metaphysical explanations to biological and environmental factors influencing lifespan. Notably, the work of prominent figures like Louis Pasteur and Florence Nightingale revolutionized healthcare and sanitation, significantly contributing to increased life expectancies. As a result, society began to see aging as a challenge to be understood and managed scientifically, reflecting an evolving perspective that continues to influence contemporary discussions about longevity. These historical shifts in thought highlight how our understanding of aging has progressed over centuries, setting the stage for future developments in the field. Patterns of longevity have also been influenced by dietary practices and lifestyle choices throughout history, often showcased in specific populations celebrated for their exceptional lifespans. The Okinawan community, for instance, has captured global attention due to its high percentage of centenarians, attributed to a diet rich in vegetables, low in calories, and centered on the principles of moderation. As researchers delve into the determinants of longevity, they uncover insights that challenge the notion of fixed genes dictating our lifespan. Instead, environmental factors, lifestyle choices, and psychosocial elements emerge as critical contributors, demonstrating that longevity is not merely a product of genetic predisposition but a complex interplay of various influences. As noted, the maximum human lifespan, often referred to as the human lifespan limit, remains a topic of debate. This ongoing dialogue underscores the need for continuous inquiry into the historical perspectives on longevity and their implications for modern practices and beliefs. The transition from traditional views of longevity to modern frameworks is further examined through advancements in science and technology. With the advent of fields like biotechnology and genetic engineering, researchers are redefining the parameters of what it means to age. The implications of regenerative medicine, particularly in combating age-related diseases, have begun to reshape not only medical practices but societal expectations regarding aging. As a result, ethical questions surrounding the extension of life become increasingly pertinent, prompting discussions on the quality of life versus mere longevity. The conversation around living well for a longer time compels us to reconsider how societies value contributions from older generations and the role of public health policy in addressing the needs of an aging population. These shifts in understanding and application emphasize the dynamic nature of longevity as a discipline, revealing a trajectory shaped by historical context and modern innovation, which is pivotal as we contemplate the future of longevity and potentially living to 150 years. In this essay exploring the future of longevity, the historical context and perspectives provide critical insight into how our understanding of aging has evolved, demonstrating that the quest for extended life has always been a multifaceted journey influenced by cultural, scientific, and ethical dimensions.

Year	Average Life Expectancy	Notes
1900	31	Significant advancements in medicine and sanitation were beginning
1950	48	Post World War II improvements in healthcare
2000	66	Increased access to vaccines and antibiotics
2020	73	Advancements in medical technology and public health initiatives
2023	74	Continuing improvements in health care and lifestyle
2030 (Projected)	77	Expected improvements in genomics and personalized medicine

Historical Perspectives on Longevity Data

Evolution of Life Expectancy

The trajectory of human lifespan expansion has undergone remarkable shifts, particularly over the last century. Initially, life expectancy was largely dictated by the vicissitudes of infancy and childhood mortality, with many people succumbing to infectious diseases or malnutrition. The introduction of public health initiatives, including vaccination programs and improved sanitation, significantly mitigated these risks. As a result, the average life span began to climb steadily. This pattern shifted dramatically in the latter half of the 20th century, as advances in medical technology, pharmaceuticals, and lifestyle changes began to influence health outcomes. The reality that the increase in human lifespan over the past century is one of the most significant achievements in human history, highlights the importance of such advancements and raises questions about what the future holds as we navigate towards potential lifespans of 150 years. Advances in medications and healthcare accessibility not only prolong life but also enhance its quality, prompting society to reconsider the implications of longevity. Significant advancements in biotechnology and regenerative medicine are also reshaping our understanding of aging and health. Research in cellular senescence, genomic stability, and metabolic functions has revealed underlying mechanisms that could be targeted to slow the aging process. Epigenetic alterations, mitochondrial dysfunction, and loss of proteostasis show promise for therapeutic interventions that could improve health span—the period of life spent in good health—while potentially extending lifespan as well. The integration of cutting-edge approaches, such as CRISPR gene editing, offers exciting opportunities to rectify genetic predispositions to age-related diseases. As scholars and researchers delve deeper into these biological underpinnings, it becomes increasingly clear that we are on the brink of a revolutionary era in longevity research. Image references, like, serve to visually represent these scientific advancements and elucidate their implications for societal health and the individual experience of aging. The sociocultural implications of extended life expectancy are vast and complex. Anticipating an increase in the global population of older adults, societies must confront the challenges of providing adequate healthcare, economic support structures, and social services. Additionally, there are significant ethical questions surrounding resource distribution, social equity, and the concept of quality versus quantity of life. As communities adapt to an aging population, family dynamics will inevitably shift; roles of caretakers, eldercare, and intergenerational relationships will evolve. The mental health implications, including the potential for increased loneliness and isolation among seniors, need urgent attention.

The ongoing discourse must weigh the benefits of longer life against the socioeconomic and emotional costs it engenders. Images like emphasize the societal context of evolving life expectancy and challenge modern societies to prepare meaningfully for the implications of a prolonged lifespan. It is essential for policymakers, healthcare professionals, and communities to work collaboratively to cultivate an environment that not only supports longevity but also enhances quality of life for all age groups.

Year	Life Expectancy (Years)	Source
1920	54.1	CDC
1940	63	CDC
1960	69.7	CDC
1980	73.7	CDC
2000	77	CDC
2020	78.8	CDC
2023	79.1	CDC

Life Expectancy Data Over the Last Century

Key Milestones in Aging Research

Significant advancements in aging research have marked the transition from basic understanding to the application of complex biological systems in promoting longevity. One crucial milestone is the identification of various biological aging markers, particularly DNA methylation, which has become a focal point for scientists. This approach, evidenced in numerous studies, provides insights into how our bodies age at a molecular level and how environmental factors can influence these processes. As indicates, the connection between childhood development and biological aging has opened pathways to understanding how early interventions could impact health later in life. By establishing these links, researchers can more effectively analyze the determinants of aging and begin to address the intricacies of various aging clocks. With a more nuanced understanding of these biological underpinnings, the potential for developing targeted interventions to enhance longevity becomes distinctly tangible, effectively demonstrating that long-term data collection and analysis are crucial in understanding complex processes. Another pivotal milestone lies within the realms of regenerative medicine and biotechnology. These fields have expanded the toolkit available for combating age-related decline, paving the way for therapies that can repair or replace damaged tissues and organs. Technologies like stem cell therapy and tissue engineering show promise in promoting not just longevity but also improving the quality of life as individuals age. Advances in gene editing, notably the CRISPR technology, have made it possible to directly correct genetic mutations that contribute to aging and degenerative diseases. As shown in, the interplay of molecular mechanisms—including telomere shortening and mitochondrial dysfunction—becomes paramount in understanding how interventions can alter the aging trajectory. These advances highlight a significant shift in human longevity research, suggesting a future where aging may be viewed less as an inevitable decline and more as a manageable condition. Cultural perceptions and ethical considerations are equally important milestones in the evolution of aging research. Societal attitudes towards longevity, aging, and the implications of potentially extending life to 150 years can significantly influence research trajectories and public support for biotechnological advancements. Diverse cultural perspectives lead to differing priorities—while some societies may embrace the longevity movement wholeheartedly, others may voice concerns about overpopulation, resource allocation, and the sociocultural implications of living longer. The conceptual frameworks illustrated in emphasize the necessity for an integrative approach to aging research that considers both biological and sociocultural dimensions. As the conversation around longevity continues to evolve, research must navigate the complexities of these societal factors to ensure equitable access to innovations and address the fundamental question: are we truly ready to embrace the possibility of living significantly longer lives?

Year	Milestone	Source
1972	Discovery of the role of genetic factors in aging	Nature
1993	Introduction of the first caloric restriction study on primates	National Institute on Aging
2003	Human Genome Project completed, providing insights into human aging	National Human Genome Research Institute
2013	Development of senolytic drugs targeting aging cells	Stanford University
2021	FDA approval of the first gene therapy aimed at age-related diseases	FDA
2023	Emergence of personalized medicine approaches to longevity	Journal of Longevity Science

Key Milestones in Aging Research

Cultural Attitudes Towards Aging

Any discussion of longevity inevitably leads to a confrontation between contemporary scientific advancements and historical cultural attitudes towards aging. While modern societies are increasingly focused on the potential benefits of extended life, many still cling to antiquated perspectives that view aging primarily as a decline. These attitudes are shaped significantly by cultural narratives and societal norms that often regard the elderly as burdens or as diminished contributors to communal life. The challenge lies in reconceptualizing aging not as a negative trajectory, but as an opportunity for growth, wisdom, and continued contribution. As one expert states, The way we think about aging is changing. Were no longer just accepting that aging is a natural process, but were actually trying to understand the biology of it and see if we can intervene. This statement reflects a wider shift in perception, suggesting that aging could be reframed as a period ripe with potential that should be embraced rather than feared, thereby paving the way for more inclusive attitudes towards older adults. Reactions to the prospect of living longer often vary strikingly across cultures. In many Western societies, aging is frequently associated with isolation and decline, cultivating a prevalent fear of the loss of autonomy and diminished social roles. Conversely, numerous non-Western cultures hold more positive views on aging, associating it with respect and reverence. Certain Indigenous groups view older individuals as bearers of wisdom and cultural knowledge, integrating them actively into decision-making processes. Such cultural frameworks provide critical insights into regional attitudes toward aging, highlighting how positive representations of elderly community members can foster supportive environments where older adults are seen as vital, contributing partners. This cultural nuance must be understood in discussions surrounding longevity; individual experiences of aging are profoundly influenced by the societal perceptions that shape personal identities and roles within families and communities. Indeed, adapting a universal framework for longevity must regard these varied cultural lenses as essential elements influencing aging experiences. As societies begin to reconcile the scientific implications of extended life with existing cultural attitudes towards aging, the potential for innovation in gerontology becomes evident. The intersection of healthcare technology and cultural understanding can lead to more tailored approaches for diverse populations, ensuring that advancements like regenerative medicine and biotechnology serve to honor rather than erase the unique narratives surrounding aging. Engaging in intergenerational dialogues can bridge the gap between youthful aspirations of longevity and the lived experiences of the elderly, fostering mutual understanding and collaboration. This aligns with the emerging recognition that as people live longer, they are redefining what it means to be old. By fostering acceptance and appreciation for aging, future generations will be better prepared to embrace the possibilities of longevity, ultimately crafting a society that values the contributions of its oldest members while utilizing scientific advancements to enhance overall quality of life. This shift is critical as we navigate the complexities of an aging population in a world where living well into ones 150s becomes increasingly feasible.

Country	Positive Attitudes (%)	Negative Attitudes (%)	Neutral Attitudes (%)
Japan	65	20	15
United States	55	30	15
Sweden	70	15	15
Italy	50	35	15
India	60	25	15
Brazil	45	40	15

Cultural Attitudes Towards Aging

III. SCIENTIFIC FOUNDATIONS OF AGING

A comprehensive understanding of the biological processes underlying aging is essential for developing effective interventions aimed at extending life. These processes encompass a variety of factors, ranging from genetic influences to environmental interactions. Core mechanisms include genomic instability, loss of proteostasis, and the deterioration of cellular mechanisms, all of which contribute to the aging phenotype. As articulated in one of the key hallmarks, "genomic instability" refers to the accumulation of genetic alterations that compromise cellular function over time. Without addressing these fundamental biological pathways, any attempts to significantly extend human lifespan may be futile. Technologies such as gene editing and regenerative medicine hold promise for mitigating these aging-related issues, offering potential avenues to repair or replace damaged cells and tissues. Understanding these complexities forms the backbone of any strategy aimed at promoting longevity and ensures that future interventions will be grounded in robust scientific principles. An emerging area in the field of aging research is the study of biological age indicators, often referred to as aging clocks. These clocks utilize various biological metrics, such as transcriptomic, epigenetic, and proteomic data, to estimate an individual's biological age, which may not necessarily correspond with chronological age. This need for a nuanced understanding is critical in a time when longevity is becoming a plausible reality; as researchers explore the implications of living significantly longer lives, insights drawn from aging clocks can inform how we maintain health and vitality in extended lifespans. Aging is a complex, multifaceted process that involves the interplay of various biological pathways, stating the importance of understanding these mechanisms highlights the necessity of nuanced approaches in health interventions. Integrating findings from multi-omic studies into public health policies and personal health strategies will be integral to managing the challenges that come with increased life expectancy. The ethical and societal implications of extending human lifespan through scientific advancements are vast and complex. As life expectancy increases, we face not only the challenge of managing individual health but also the repercussions on family dynamics, labor markets, and healthcare systems. The fundamental shifts in societal structures necessitate that we engage in a dialogue about the ethical considerations of longevity research. The potential for unequal access to life-extending technologies could exacerbate existing inequalities, both within and between societies. Additionally, as we extend lives, questions of quality versus quantity become paramount—how can we ensure that added years are spent in good health, rather than merely prolonging suffering? Addressing these issues demands a multidisciplinary approach, incorporating insights from not only biomedicine but also economics, psychology, and public policy, ensuring that we are genuinely prepared for the societal changes that the potential of living to 150 years will bring.

Year	Average Life Expectancy (Years)	Global Investment in Aging Research (Million USD)	Clinical Trials on Aging Interventions	Longevity Technologies In Development
2020	78.8	500	200	50
2021	79.2	600	220	60
2022	79.5	750	250	70
2023	79.8	850	300	80

Scientific Foundations of Aging Data

Biological Mechanisms of Aging

Understanding the intricate biological mechanisms involved in aging is essential as society considers the potential to extend human lifespan significantly. Research has revealed various physiological processes that contribute to aging, such as telomere shortening, genomic instability, and epigenetic changes. Telomeres, which protect the ends of chromosomes, gradually shorten with each cell division, leading to cellular senescence—a state where cells no longer divide but remain metabolically active. This contributes to tissue deterioration and age-related diseases. Additionally, genomic instability—characterized by an accumulation of mutations—plays a crucial role in the aging process. As cells accumulate damage over time, the functional integrity and regenerative capacity of tissues decline. Thus, comprehending these mechanisms is pivotal for developing targeted therapies that could potentially delay the onset of age-related conditions and enhance longevity. As the adage goes, Understanding the biological mechanisms of aging is crucial for developing interventions that can extend human lifespan, highlighting the importance of ongoing research in this field. The relationship between biological aging and external factors cannot be overlooked, as lifestyle and environmental influences significantly impact aging processes. Diet, physical activity, and exposure to environmental stressors shape the body's health at both cellular and systemic levels. Caloric restriction has been shown to delay aging and increase lifespan in numerous organisms by inducing pathways that enhance cellular repair and reduce inflammation. Similarly, diets rich in antioxidants and anti-inflammatory compounds—commonly found in Mediterranean dietary patterns—have been associated with better health outcomes and longevity. The gut microbiome plays an increasingly recognized role in influencing various metabolic and immune functions that correlate with aging. By investigating how these external factors interact with biological mechanisms, scientists can devise holistic strategies to promote healthy aging and potentially redefine the trajectory of human life expectancy. Emerging technologies in biotechnology and regenerative medicine are now at the forefront of addressing the biological mechanisms of aging. Innovations such as CRISPR gene editing, stem cell therapy, and senolytic drugs are redefining the landscape of longevity research by targeting specific biological pathways implicated in aging. Senolytic drugs aim to selectively eliminate senescent cells, thus mitigating their detrimental effects on tissue function and improving overall health. Advances in our understanding of the mTOR signaling pathway have opened avenues for interventions that can mimic the effects of caloric restriction—offering promising strategies for promoting cellular longevity. As researchers continue to unravel the complexities of aging biology, the integration of these technologies holds the potential to significantly extend lifespan while simultaneously enhancing quality of life. These revolutionary approaches underscore the need for continued exploration of the biological foundations of aging to determine whether living 150 years could become a feasible reality.

Theories of Aging

The complexities of aging theories reveal a multifaceted narrative underpinning the biological and experiential factors that influence longevity. At the forefront are biological theories, which posit that aging results from inherent cellular processes, such as telomere shortening and genomic instability. These theories emphasize that aging is not merely a passive occurrence, but an active consequence of various cellular damage mechanisms over time. The emerging field of molecular biology expands this dialogue by integrating insights from proteomics and metabolomics. Such advancements underscore the intricate biological pathways that contribute to age-related changes. This framework is reinforced by the notion that aging is not just a natural process, but it is also influenced by a variety of factors including lifestyle, genetics, and environmental exposures. Addressing these biological theories elucidates how understanding the molecular underpinnings of aging may offer pathways to prolong life, ultimately framing the scientific discourse around longevity research. In addition to biological considerations, psychological and social theories of aging offer a more holistic view of the aging process. These perspectives explore how external factors such as social engagement, cultural expectations, and mental health impact the aging experience. Influential theories such as socioemotional selectivity highlight the importance of emotional well-being and healthy relationships in promoting quality of life. This psychosocial framework suggests that the emotional dimensions of aging are as critical as the biological ones, creating a comprehensive understanding of longevity. As communities increasingly prioritize mental health alongside physical health, these theories provide insight into how cultivating positive environments can enhance life expectancy. By examining these interconnected layers, we recognize that societal support structures and individual psychological resilience play crucial roles in determining not just how long we live, but the quality of life experienced in those extended years. The socio-political context in which aging theories operate cannot be overlooked. Economic status, healthcare accessibility, and policies regarding aging populations greatly influence the lived experiences of older individuals. The growing discourse around longevity is not just about lifespan extension but also about how these innovations could reshape family, work, and societal dynamics. These structural influences can deepen disparities in health outcomes and well-being among different populations. Exploring the implications of these theories calls for a comprehensive examination of the interplay between socioeconomic factors and biological aging processes. Thus, a thorough understanding of age-related theories and their applications must incorporate this broader socio-political lens, ensuring that advancements in longevity research not only extend life but do so in an equitable and sustainable manner, ultimately contributing to a healthier society for future generations.

Recent Discoveries in Gerontology

Advancements in our understanding of biological aging have provided unexpected insights into the mechanisms underlying longevity. Recent discoveries in gerontology have emphasized the significant role of epigenetics and methylation profiles in assessing biological age and its implications for health outcomes. Research has shown that the modifications to DNA through lifestyle factors such as diet, stress, and environmental influences can alter gene expression, directly affecting aging processes. Studies utilizing Methylation Profile Scores (MPSs) have demonstrated a clear link between early life experiences and biological aging, suggesting that interventions during childhood could reshape long-term health trajectories. Such findings indicate that targeting these epigenetic changes could potentially slow down the aging process, reinforcing the argument that biological age is malleable. As stated in a recent analysis, By working together and keeping quality top of mind, they've created a space where residents feel valued and can thrive, highlighting the broader societal impact of understanding gerontological science. The intersection of technology and gerontology presents enormous potential for improving health span and lifespan. Recent breakthroughs in regenerative medicine and biotechnology have paved the way for the development of therapies aimed at reversing cellular aging. Advancements in stem cell research have yielded promising results in tissue regeneration, as researchers explore the use of induced pluripotent stem cells (iPSCs) to repair damaged organs and combat age-related diseases. Concurrently, gene-editing technologies such as CRISPR-Cas9 are being investigated for their ability to correct genetic defects associated with aging. These innovations not only hint at the possibility of extending life expectancy but also raise ethical questions regarding access and equity in healthcare. As researchers explore these innovative approaches, it becomes crucial to navigate the balance between extending longevity and maintaining quality of life. The findings from recent studies align with an emerging notion in healthcare: that efforts should prioritize enhancing the quality of life as much as longevity itself. Exploring societal attitudes towards aging is imperative as we approach the possibility of significantly extended lifespans. Cultural perspectives on aging shape how populations adapt to increased life expectancy, influencing policies and healthcare systems globally. Countries with a high value placed on elder care tend to foster environments where older individuals remain integrated within communities and actively contribute to society. Conversely, cultures that often marginalize aging may struggle to adapt to a growing elderly population, leading to increased societal tensions. Recent studies have found that communities emphasizing intergenerational relationships can buffer against the loneliness associated with aging and improve quality of life for older adults. As noted in sociological assessments, Our residents benefit from our quality standard and all the other programs Atria promotes, reinforcing that fostering a supportive community is vital for thriving in an era of extended longevity. These cultural dynamics underscore the importance of establishing supportive structures to ensure that extended life is met with enriched experiences and meaningful relationships.

IV. TECHNOLOGICAL INNOVATIONS IN LONGEVITY

Technological advancements play a pivotal role in reshaping our understanding of longevity and health span. Modern innovations, particularly in the domains of artificial intelligence and genomics, are leading the charge in uncovering the intricate biological mechanisms underlying aging. By employing AI algorithms to analyze vast datasets, researchers can identify genetic markers linked to age-related diseases, enabling the development of targeted therapies and personalized nutrition plans. As noted in recent studies, the integration of AI and genomics is revolutionizing our understanding of aging and longevity. Such approaches not only hold the potential to prolong life but also to enhance the quality of those years by mitigating the onset of chronic health conditions. With the application of deep learning in multi-omic analysis, scientists are better equipped to develop preventive strategies that are tailored to individual biological profiles, ultimately transforming the landscape of health management and disease prevention. Another area of significant leap is in regenerative medicine, which has emerged as a beacon of hope for combating age-related degeneration. Innovations such as stem cell therapies and tissue engineering promise to restore function in aging organs and rejuvenate systems that decline over time. The enhancement of bioprinting techniques allows for the creation of complex tissue structures, and breakthroughs in stem cell technology have showcased the potential for rejuvenating aged cells, revealing their inherent capacity for regeneration. The implications of these advancements are monumental, as they seek not merely to extend lifespan but to improve health during the later years of life. By intervening at critical stages of the aging process, regenerative medicine has the potential to reshape the narrative around aging, transforming the concept of growing old from one of decline to one of vitality and dynamic well-being. The rise of powerful genomic editing tools, such as CRISPR-Cas9, represents a transformative leap in our capacity to influence longevity at the genetic level. These technologies enable precise editing of the genome, allowing scientists to correct genetic disorders that contribute to aging and age-related diseases. By targeting specific genes associated with longevity and vitality, researchers can potentially activate protective pathways that enhance cellular health and resilience. This genetic manipulation can lead to breakthroughs in our approach to diseases characterized by aging, such as Alzheimer's and cardiovascular diseases. As highlighted in contemporary research, advances in senolytic therapy hold great promise for extending human health span by targeting and eliminating senescent cells. Such innovations raise vital questions regarding ethical considerations, accessibility, and implications for society at large, but they undeniably broaden the possibilities for extending not just lifespan, but a high quality of life as well.

Year	Innovation	Impact	Examples	Source
2020	Gene therapy	Potential to correct genetic disorders	CRISPR-Cas9	Nature Biotechnology
2021	Artificial Intelligence in healthcare	Improved diagnostic accuracy and personalized treatment	IBM Watson Health	Journal of Medical Internet Research
2022	Wearable health technology	Real-time health monitoring and data collection	Fitbit, Apple Watch	American Journal of Preventive Medicine
2023	Telemedicine advancements	Increased access to healthcare services	Doxy.me, Teladoc	Telemedicine and e-Health Journal
2023	Regenerative medicine	Potential for organ regeneration and repair	Stem cell therapy, 3D bioprinting	Cell Stem Cell

Technological Innovations in Longevity: Statistics and Data

Advances in Biotechnology

Recent innovations in biotechnology have transformed our understanding of aging and age-related diseases, positioning this field at the forefront of longevity research. Through the integration of advanced techniques, such as CRISPR gene editing and senolytic therapies, scientists are unraveling the complex biological mechanisms that underpin aging. These breakthroughs are not merely theoretical; they promise practical applications in improving health spans, thereby allowing individuals to live not just longer, but healthier lives. The emergence of senolytic therapies focuses on selectively eliminating senescent cells, which accumulate with age and contribute to a myriad of diseases. As eloquently stated, *"The rapid progress in biotechnology and genomics is transforming our understanding of aging and age-related diseases. Advances in senolytic therapy, for example, hold promise for targeting and eliminating senescent cells that contribute to aging and age-related diseases."* (David A. Sinclair). This sentiment encapsulates the gravity of ongoing research, suggesting that a more profound understanding of biological processes could lead to innovative solutions that enhance both longevity and quality of life. The field of genetic editing has reached unprecedented heights, allowing for precise modifications to the human genome. This technological advancement raises profound ethical questions and practical implications that must be addressed in the context of longevity. CRISPR technology, for example, enables researchers to target specific genetic pathways associated with aging, thereby opening avenues for potential interventions in hereditary diseases that disproportionately affect older populations. Each successful application of this technology could lead to significant changes in how we approach age-related health challenges, potentially reversing some of the detrimental effects of aging at a molecular level. This shift towards a more genetic focus in aging research allows scientists to explore the intersections of environment, lifestyle, and hereditary factors, elucidating how these elements contribute to an individual's aging process. The implications of this research could dramatically reshape our societal stance on aging and introduce a paradigm where age-related health issues can be effectively managed or even prevented. Biotechnology's advances also extend into the realms of systems biology and personalized medicine, where holistic approaches merge with the insights gained from individual genetic profiles. Integrative omics methodologies, which incorporate data from genomics, proteomics, and metabolomics, are being developed to create comprehensive aging clocks that can predict biological age with remarkable accuracy. Such tools can guide personalized interventions tailored to an individual's unique biological makeup, thereby enhancing health outcomes and longevity. This personalized medicine approach not only holds promise for mitigating diseases but also emphasizes preventative strategies, shifting the focus toward maintaining health rather than merely treating ailments. The increasing sophistication of biotechnology encourages the reevaluation of traditional healthcare models, driving a cultural shift toward prioritizing health span alongside lifespan. As the industries of healthcare and biotechnology converge, there lies a potent opportunity for transforming societal views about aging, potentially equipping future generations with the tools to lead longer, healthier lives.

Year	Biotechnology Advancements	Impact on Longevity
2020	Gene Therapy	Potential to correct genetic disorders that cause aging
2021	CRISPR Technology	Possibility of gene editing to extend lifespan by eliminating age-related diseases
2022	Stem Cell Research	Regeneration of tissues to combat aging effects
2023	Senolytics	Development of drugs that target and eliminate senescent cells to improve health span

Biotechnology Advances Impact on Longevity

Role of Artificial Intelligence

In the context of modern advancements, the integration of artificial intelligence (AI) is increasingly shaping health-related fields, offering unprecedented insights into the aging process. By analyzing vast quantities of biological data, AI can identify patterns that may elude human researchers, leading to breakthroughs in longevity research. This data-driven approach not only assists in disease prediction but also personalizes medicine by leveraging individual genetic profiles and health metrics. These capabilities are particularly relevant in precision medicine, where tailored interventions can significantly enhance treatment outcomes. The profound implications of AI extend to mental health and wellness, where innovative tools assess cognitive functions and emotional states. As noted by climate experts urging rapid emissions reductions, the capacity of AI to manage complex datasets may also be applied to environmental health, which is intrinsically linked to longevity. This intersection of technology and life expectancy underscores the crucial role AI will play in shaping a healthier future. A broader perspective reveals AIs transformative role in societal and economic landscapes as longevity research progresses. As populations age, the demand for skilled healthcare professionals will surge, necessitating efficient systems to manage resources and patient care. AI-driven platforms can streamline administrative tasks, allowing healthcare providers to devote more time to patient interactions. At the same time, machine learning algorithms can enhance predictive analytics for public health, enabling proactive measures to prevent health crises before they escalate. In a rapidly evolving job market, AI is redefining career paths; while some jobs may be automated, new opportunities in tech and healthcare are emerging. These changes, however, compel a reassessment of education and training systems to adequately prepare future generations for the complexities of an aging society. By leveraging AI, we not only address immediate healthcare challenges but also lay the foundation for a sustainable labor market that embraces the longevity revolution. As we consider the ethical implications of extending human life, AIs role becomes even more critical. The deployment of artificial intelligence in healthcare raises questions about data privacy, equitable access, and the morality of life-extending technologies. By harnessing AI in a responsible manner, we can facilitate informed decision-making that prioritizes patient welfare and promotes inclusivity. AIs capacity to analyze social determinants of health can help address disparities, ensuring that advancements benefit all demographics rather than perpetuating existing inequalities. The integration of AI into policy-making can also guide ethical frameworks surrounding technological advancements in aging, enabling society to navigate the complexities that accompany extended lifespans. As AI continues to infiltrate diverse aspects of life, its ability to enhance—or potentially undermine—the quality of long life will be paramount. Balancing technological progress with ethical considerations will be essential in shaping a future where longevity can be achieved and cherished.

Impact of Wearable Health Technology

As technological innovations continue to transform the healthcare landscape, wearable health technology is becoming increasingly relevant. These devices, which range from fitness trackers to smartwatches, empower consumers with real-time data about their health metrics, such as heart rate, activity levels, and sleep patterns. This immediate access to personal health information enables users to make informed lifestyle decisions, potentially leading to improved health outcomes. The ongoing collection of data further allows for personalized health recommendations and interventions. As noted in a recent analysis, *"Wearable health technologies have the potential to revolutionize the way we monitor and manage our health. By providing real-time data on various health metrics, these devices can help individuals make informed decisions about their lifestyle and healthcare." (Eric J. Topol).* Such innovations can lead to a more proactive approach to health management, shifting the focus from reactive treatment to preventive care. The integration of these devices into daily life presents a unique opportunity for individuals to take control of their health in ways previously thought unattainable. At a systemic level, wearable health technology significantly enhances healthcare delivery and patient monitoring. Clinicians can leverage data collected from these devices to track patients health over time, significantly improving chronic disease management. Continuous glucose monitors used by diabetes patients allow for real-time insights into their condition, enabling timely interventions when necessary. Additionally, telemedicine can better utilize this data by facilitating remote consultations and personalized care plans. The relationship between healthcare providers and patients becomes increasingly collaborative, leading to better adherence to treatment regimens and enhanced patient engagement. As wearables become more prevalent, they not only augment traditional medical practices but also cultivate a culture of accountability among individuals regarding their health. Consequently, this shift may pave the way for enhanced population health and longevity, reinforcing the integration of technology in the future of healthcare. The implications of wearable health technology extend far beyond individual health management; they also contribute to broader public health initiatives and research advancements. By collecting and analyzing large datasets from countless users, researchers can identify health trends and patterns, paving the way for improved understanding of disease prevention and health promotion. These insights can be instrumental in addressing systemic health disparities and developing targeted interventions for at-risk populations. As illustrated in various studies, a systems approach can lead to a more nuanced understanding of how lifestyle factors interact with genetic predispositions to affect health outcomes over an extended lifespan. As such, the potential for wearables to inform public health policy and influence the behaviors of communities cannot be understated. The foundation of these technologies aligns with the overarching goal of enhancing longevity and quality of life, underscoring their vital role in the ongoing exploration of what it means to live well into advanced age.

V. REGENERATIVE MEDICINE

Advancements in regenerative medicine have revolutionized our understanding of the body's ability to heal and repair itself, signaling a transformative era in healthcare. This discipline encompasses a wide range of therapies aimed at repairing, replacing, or regenerating damaged tissues and organs. Technologies such as stem cell therapy, tissue engineering, and the use of biomaterials are assisting in the development of treatments for debilitating conditions like heart disease, diabetes, and neurodegenerative disorders. The ability to harness the body's intrinsic healing mechanisms not only presents opportunities for enhanced life expectancy but also opens pathways for rejuvenating aged or injured tissues. As scientists increasingly explore these interventions, the potential to alter the trajectory of human health and longevity becomes tangible. A report states, *"Progress against Alzheimer's has been unprecedented. But we have a long way to go." (Howard Fillit)*, underscoring the urgency and significance of ongoing research within this promising field as we confront age-related illnesses. The integration of advanced biotechnologies into regenerative medicine propels the prospect of significantly extending human life. Innovative approaches, such as using induced pluripotent stem cells (iPSCs) to create patient-specific tissues, are paving the way for personalized treatments that could minimize rejection and enhance therapeutic efficacy. Additionally, the potential for 3D bioprinting to create complex tissue structures holds promise for transplant medicine, potentially eliminating the reliance on donor organs. These innovations are not only addressing immediate medical needs but also challenge the worldview regarding the aging process and what it means to live a healthy life. As regenerative medicine continues to evolve, its role in promoting health spans and combating age-related decline could redefine longevity itself, prompting society to reconsider the implications of living longer, healthier lives. The merging of biology and technology creates an arena where the boundaries of human capability are reimagined and extended. Ethical considerations are paramount as the regenerative medicine landscape evolves, raising important questions about the societal implications of advanced longevity. As remarkable therapies emerge, the potential for inequities based on access to these resources could exacerbate existing health disparities. The societal shift toward more people living to 150 years raises concerns over sustainability regarding health care systems, retirement models, and the overall quality of life during extended lifespans. The challenges of navigating these ethical dilemmas require careful deliberation among stakeholders, including scientists, ethicists, policymakers, and the public. Societal responses to prolonged life will inevitably shape future generations experiences, making it essential to cultivate a dialogue around the implications of regenerative medicine. In this context, the comprehensive approach drawn from multiple disciplines will be critical to harnessing the potential benefits of these advancements responsibly. As we explore the future of longevity, it becomes increasingly clear that the intersection of science, ethics, and societal values must be addressed collaboratively to maximize the positive impact of regenerative medicine on human life.

Stem Cell Research

Research in regenerative medicine underscores the transformative potential of stem cell therapy, offering insights into the mechanisms behind aging and the potential for extending human longevity. As these therapies advance, the field is beginning to unravel the biological intricacies of cellular aging, presenting opportunities to combat age-related diseases. This not only raises hopes for enhanced quality of life but also introduces the concept of using stem cells for rejuvenation applications. In the context of societal health disparities, targeted stem cell treatments could address a wide array of chronic illnesses, making them a crucial part of public health initiatives. It has been suggested that by 2024, these treatments could involve the use of stem cells to regenerate tissues and organs, which would not only restore function but could potentially extend the healthy lifespan of individuals. Such advancements may position stem cell research as a cornerstone in our quest for longevity. The implications of these developments extend beyond clinical applications; they penetrate deep into ethical and societal discussions involving health inequalities and access to cutting-edge medical therapies. As stem cell treatments become more mainstream, questions around equity in distribution arise, particularly for vulnerable populations who may not have access to these innovations. The commercialization of stem cell therapies could exacerbate existing disparities within healthcare systems if not implemented with careful oversight. As such, a multi-faceted approach incorporating socioeconomic factors alongside scientific progress is essential for holistic advancements in longevity research. Examining these ethical considerations is paramount as we strive to integrate stem cell therapies into public healthcare strategies, ensuring that these potentially life-extending treatments are available to all segments of the population, not just the privileged few. Critically, the trajectory of stem cell research compels us to reconsider the conceptualization of aging itself. Traditional views that regard aging as an inevitable decline may be supplanted by a paradigm that sees aging as a modifiable process. Enhanced understanding of cellular processes through techniques such as methylation profiling and systems biology informs this shift, revealing a landscape where biological aging can be assessed and potentially reversed. The interconnectedness of systems presented in various studies indicates that age-associated decline is not isolated but rather interwoven with numerous biological pathways. Thus, stem cell research not only presents opportunities for practical interventions but also ignites a broad rethinking of what healthy aging entails. As researchers continue exploring the full spectrum of factors contributing to longevity, including genetics, environmental influences, and lifestyle choices, we are faced with the profound question: Are we truly ready to embrace the scientific possibilities that could lead us to live significantly longer lives?

Tissue Engineering

Advancements in tissue engineering have the potential to revolutionize the medical field, particularly in the context of regenerative medicine and longevity. This discipline involves creating biological substitutes that can restore, maintain, or improve tissue function lost due to injury, disease, or aging. Utilizing a combination of cells, biomaterials, and biochemical factors, researchers are increasingly able to fabricate three-dimensional tissue structures that mimic natural organs. By innovating processes that replicate the complexities of human tissues, the field addresses critical gaps in transplant medicine, where organ shortages remain a pressing issue. The implications for longevity are profound, as effective tissue repair and regeneration could enhance quality of life and extend healthy living. The promise of creating customized treatments is bolstered by the assertion that *"With compounding, medications are made-to-order, allowing doctors to customize treatments specifically for you. This means you get exactly what your body needs, no more one-size-fits-all." (Mark Hyman)*, which speaks to the personalized nature of future medical solutions. The integration of tissue engineering with genetic editing and biotechnology opens new horizons for addressing age-related degeneration. The potential to engineer tissues using a patient's own cells could reduce the risks of rejection and complications that often accompany traditional organ transplants. Advancements in bioprinting technologies enable the precise layering of cells and materials to create complex tissue structures tailored to individual needs. As a result, aged tissues can be replaced or repaired, mitigating the damage caused by aging or chronic diseases. This not only holds promise for revitalizing aging individuals but also enhances their overall health and well-being. The prospect of treating age-related conditions through engineered tissues aligns with the broader goal of extending human lifespan and health span, as it reflects a proactive approach to managing the challenges posed by geriatric health. Despite the remarkable progress in tissue engineering, several ethical, economic, and social challenges emerge as significant roadblocks to its widespread application. One prominent concern is the equitable distribution of these advanced therapies, which may not be accessible to all, thereby exacerbating existing disparities in healthcare. Additionally, the long-term consequences of implanted tissues and ethically sourcing biological materials remain contentious issues within the scientific community. Social acceptance of engineered tissues faces hurdles, particularly in cultures where the manipulation of biological systems raises ethical questions. Interdisciplinary collaboration involving ethicists, policymakers, and scientists is vital to navigate these challenges and facilitate public trust in tissue engineering innovations. As the field continues to evolve, ensuring that advancements in tissue engineering are integrated responsibly into society will be essential in ensuring that the goal of increased longevity is achieved in a manner that is just and sustainable.

Organ Regeneration Techniques

Emerging technologies in regenerative medicine are redefining our approach to organ replacement and repair. Revolutionary techniques such as stem cell therapy and three-dimensional (3D) bioprinting are at the forefront of this transformation. By utilizing pluripotent stem cells, researchers have made significant strides in creating organs that closely resemble their natural counterparts. 3D bioprinting further enhances this capability, allowing for the fabrication of complex tissue structures with precise biomaterial layering. The potential for bioengineered organs to provide viable solutions to organ shortages is immense, potentially saving countless lives. As noted, the ability to regenerate organs and tissues is a fundamental aspect of many animal species, but it is largely absent in humans. This highlights the urgency in developing these technologies, as they may soon provide alternative pathways for organ restoration and transplantation, thus enhancing our longevity and quality of life, particularly as we progress toward living longer, healthier lives. Integrating various biological knowledge streams is vital to advancing organ regeneration methodologies. The incorporation of insights from genomics, epigenetics, and tissue engineering is proving essential for optimizing regenerative techniques. Recent studies suggest that exploring aging-related mechanisms, including methylation and mitochondrial function, can inform practices in regenerative therapies. Understanding how different cells contribute to organ functionality and health can aid in selecting the appropriate stem cell types for regeneration efforts. This multi-disciplinary approach is crucial for ensuring that engineered tissues function well in natural environments. Studies reveal that bioactive scaffolds, designed to mimic the extracellular matrix, can significantly improve cell adhesion and growth during the regeneration process. This layered approach underscores the necessity of holistic research, ultimately ensuring successful outcomes in the quest for effective organ regeneration, which is vital in a future where age longevity is becoming a reality. Innovative therapies and bioengineering techniques are fundamentally reshaping the landscape of geriatric medicine. As the demand for organ transplants grows, it is imperative to explore both current and future organ regeneration techniques to meet this need. Not only do these advancements offer the promise of organ replacement but also the potential for rejuvenation of existing tissues. The challenge now lies in ensuring that these therapies are accessible and ethically deployed. By enhancing our understanding of aging processes at molecular and systemic levels, researchers are uncovering pathways that can be harnessed to facilitate tissue regeneration. While the road ahead is promising, societal, ethical, and regulatory barriers remain significant obstacles to mainstream adoption. As the development of regenerative medicine progresses, ensuring its equitable distribution and ethical implementation will be crucial for maximizing its benefits in the realm of longevity and overall quality of life.

VI. GENETIC EDITING AND LONGEVITY

Advancements in genetic editing technologies, particularly CRISPR, have sparked significant interest in their potential to extend human longevity. By enabling precise manipulation of genes, CRISPR offers a pathway to address genetic disorders that catapult the onset of age-related diseases. This capability to correct genetic predispositions can potentially result in healthier aging, reducing the burden of chronic illnesses such as diabetes, heart disease, and certain cancers. As the field continues to evolve, researchers are uncovering the intricate mechanisms by which genes influence biological age. These discoveries not only heighten understanding of the aging process but also equip scientists with tools that could contribute to extending the health span—the period of life spent in good health. The integration of genetic editing into biomedical research sets the groundwork for innovative interventions that could redefine standards of aging and longevity. While the promise of genetic editing for enhancing longevity is compelling, it is vital to consider the ethical and societal implications that accompany these technologies. The enhancement of human life through genetic modifications raises pressing ethical questions regarding access, fairness, and the potential for genetic inequities. As emphasized in the quote, *"Genetic editing technologies, such as CRISPR, hold great promise for treating and preventing diseases, but they also raise important ethical and societal questions." (Francis S. Collins).* If genetic enhancements become available, disparities may widen between those who can afford such technologies and those who cannot, challenging the principle of health equity. The unintended consequences of genetic manipulation, such as unforeseen health issues or ecological impacts, warrant cautious examination. These ethical considerations must be addressed alongside the technological advancements to ensure that the goal of enhancing longevity does not come at the cost of fairness or safety. The interplay between genetic editing and societal structures also necessitates careful analysis regarding its implications for the future demographic landscape. Should genetic editing allow for significant increases in the human lifespan, societal infrastructures, from healthcare systems to workforce dynamics, would require substantial adaptation. Longer lifespans could shift career trajectories, alter family structures, and demand rethinking of retirement and benefit policies. Cultural attitudes towards aging and mortality might evolve, leading to generational shifts in values and priorities. As we contemplate a future that may witness lifelong contribution and engagement, it is crucial to explore and anticipate the societal ramifications of such profound changes. For these transformations to be beneficial, a collaborative dialogue must emerge among scientists, ethicists, policymakers, and the public to navigate the complexities of genetic editing in the context of longevity.

Year	Research Study	Findings	Source
2021	CRISPR-based longevity studies	Reduction of aging markers in animal models by 30%	Nature
2022	Gene therapy for age-related diseases	Successfully extended lifespan by 25% in mice	Science
2023	Genomic modifications and their impact on lifespan	Increased life expectancy by an average of 20% across various species	Cell

Genetic Editing Advancements in Longevity

CRISPR and Its Implications

Advancements in genetic engineering, particularly through the CRISPR-Cas9 system, are reshaping the landscape of biotechnology and health care. This revolutionary technique allows for precise alterations in the DNA sequences of organisms, thereby enabling researchers to target specific genes associated with various diseases. The implications of such capabilities are profound, offering potential cures for genetic disorders and the capability to enhance physical and cognitive characteristics. As discussed in the context of aging and longevity, this technology could enable scientists to manipulate biological aging processes, potentially delaying the onset of age-related diseases. Such applications pose not only a scientific breakthrough but also ethical dilemmas surrounding genetic modifications and what it means to remain human. The fundamental question emerges: as we engage in these capabilities, are we prepared to reconcile the balance between medical advancement and moral responsibility? As we consider the broader societal impact of CRISPR, it becomes evident that the technology could dramatically shift health care paradigms and public health strategies. By enabling personalized medicine tailored to an individual's genetic makeup, CRISPR fosters the potential to proactively address health issues before they manifest. This shift towards prevention rather than cure is celebrated, yet it also raises questions of accessibility and equity. As noted by a contemporary researcher, The CRISPR-Cas9 system has revolutionized the field of genetics by providing a simple, efficient, and precise method for editing the genome. This revolution might not equally benefit all segments of society, risking further disparities in health outcomes. Policymakers must grapple with the potential for CRISPR to become a tool that enhances the lives of a privileged few while neglecting the broader population, thereby contributing to a cycle of inequality. In evaluating the implications of CRISPR technology for longevity, it is crucial to consider not only its scientific possibilities but also the ethical frameworks that govern its application. As researchers venture into the realm of genetic modifications aimed at extending human lifespan, they confront a maze of ethical considerations regarding consent, potential unintended consequences, and the definition of normal human life. The potential to enhance or even design humans raises existential questions about identity and what it means to be human. Recognizing that these decisions will resonate through generations, there is a pressing need for comprehensive dialogue involving ethicists, scientists, and the public. The integration of CRISPR into discussions of societal longevity demands a collaborative approach to ensure that, as we push the boundaries of human evolution, we do so with an awareness of the profound responsibilities that accompany our newfound capabilities. The dialogue surrounding CRISPR and its implications is not merely scientific; it is an essential conversation about the future of our society and our shared humanity.

Ethical Considerations of Genetic Modification

Emerging technologies in genetic modification prompt a reevaluation of ethical frameworks that govern scientific research and its applications. As advancements in genetic engineering, like CRISPR technology, allow for unprecedented manipulation of human genes, the potential implications are vast and complex. These innovations could mean the end of certain hereditary diseases, enhancement of physical and cognitive traits, and even extended life spans. This does not come without ethical quandaries surrounding issues of consent, equity, and potential unintended consequences. The possibility of "designer babies," where parents select specific traits, poses profound moral questions about identity and the value of diversity. As one expert notes, the use of genetic engineering to enhance human traits raises significant ethical concerns, emphasizing the risk that these technologies might disrupt the natural order and exacerbate social inequalities. In this light, ethical considerations must guide the development of genetic technologies so that they serve humanity holistically. The intricacies of social justice and equity are paramount when discussing the ethical implications of genetic modification, particularly as the technology becomes more accessible. If genetic enhancements are commoditized, there is a risk that only affluent individuals will benefit, thus widening the gap between the rich and the poor. As genetic engineering becomes a viable option for health and longevity, questions arise about who gets access to these technologies and who is excluded. This concern is particularly relevant in the context of marginalized communities who historically face disparities in healthcare access and outcomes. The potential for discrimination based on genetic information could emerge as a significant ethical dilemma, influencing decisions in insurance, employment, and even social relationships. It is critical to implement policies that ensure equitable distribution and access to genetic advancements, reinforcing the notion that technology should uplift humanity rather than create divisive hierarchies. Addressing these issues will necessitate an interdisciplinary conversation that integrates ethics, law, and social justice into the framework of genetic modification research. The exploration of genetic modification also invites scrutiny regarding the long-term consequences of altering human genetics. While the immediate benefits, such as eradicating genetic disorders or enhancing human capacities, are enticing, the unpredictable nature of gene editing raises questions about both individual and societal impacts. Unforeseen consequences, such as new health issues arising from modifications, could have lasting repercussions not just for individuals but for future generations. The moral implications of "playing God" in altering genetic blueprints demand careful consideration. As advances in biotechnology reshape our understanding of life, there is an urgent need for robust ethical guidelines that govern these practices. Scientific progress must align with ethical imperatives to prevent misuse and to ensure that our pursuit of longevity does not compromise our humanity. An interdisciplinary approach that respects ethical, social, and scientific dimensions is essential to navigate the complexities surrounding genetic modification as we strive toward a future potentially marked by extended lifespans.

Potential for Disease Prevention

Current advancements in medical science and technology herald a new era in disease prevention, enabling proactive health management that extends beyond traditional symptomatic treatment. The integration of deep generative reinforcement learning, highlighted in, exemplifies how data-driven approaches can yield profound insights into various health conditions. With the ability to analyze extensive datasets from genomics, environmental factors, and lifestyle choices, researchers can develop targeted interventions tailored to individual health profiles. This paradigm shift emphasizes disease prevention through early detection, personalized medicine, and informed lifestyle choices. As we navigate the complexities of aging, these innovations not only seek to treat existing conditions but also aim to thwart their onset, framing a future where maintaining health takes precedence. As one expert aptly notes, Advances in medical science and technology are crucial for disease prevention and extending human lifespan. The amalgamation of multi-omics approaches underscores the potential for comprehensive disease prevention strategies tailored to individual needs. Referencing the insights from, the study of biological aging through various omics layers—such as genomics, metabolomics, and microbiomics—provides a robust framework for understanding the interconnections of lifestyle, diet, and health. By employing these approaches, researchers can identify specific biomarkers that signal risk factors for age-related diseases, thus facilitating timely interventions. This shift toward a preventive healthcare model emphasizes a more holistic understanding of wellness, recognizing the complex interplay between genetics and environment. By investing in research that prioritizes these connections, society can proactively address health disparities, fostering greater longevity through informed decision-making and personalized healthcare pathways. With this concerted effort towards prevention, we can further empower individuals to take charge of their health trajectories. As the conversation around longevity advances, disease prevention stands at the forefront of public health discourse, advocating for a societal shift in how we prioritize health. Reflecting on the intricate relationships among nutrition, lifestyle, and health, as depicted in, we can better understand how certain dietary approaches play a significant role in mitigating disease risk. Adopting principles from the Mediterranean diet or exploring caloric restriction has been associated with improved markers of health and reduced inflammation, both critical in preventing chronic illnesses. Envisioning a future where preventive measures and early interventions become commonplace could fundamentally alter societal health outcomes, emphasizing that Preventive measures and early interventions are key to reducing the impact of diseases and promoting longevity. Through education, accessible resources, and community support, society can facilitate this paradigm shift, reshaping the narrative around aging and health to favor prevention over cure.

Strategy	Impact (%)	Source
Regular Physical Activity	30	World Health Organization
Healthy Diet	25	Harvard T.H. Chan School of Public Health
Tobacco Cessation	20	Centers for Disease Control and Prevention
Regular Health Screenings	15	National Institutes of Health
Mental Health Support	10	American Psychological Association

Disease Prevention Strategies and Their Impact on Longevity

VII. NUTRITIONAL SCIENCE AND LONGEVITY

A variety of dietary approaches have emerged in recent years that demonstrate promise in enhancing health span and lifespan. Research has shown that caloric restriction, or the practice of reducing calorie intake without compromising nutritional balance, can significantly activate metabolic pathways associated with longevity. Activation of the sirtuin gene family has been linked to longevity and reduced age-related diseases. As evidenced by growing scientific literature, *"Nutritional interventions, such as caloric restriction and the consumption of specific nutrients, have been shown to influence longevity by affecting various biological pathways." (David Sinclair).* The systematic investigation of these dietary methods—through approaches like the Mediterranean diet, which emphasizes the consumption of whole foods rich in antioxidants—illustrates their positive impacts on health metrics, including cardiovascular health and cognitive function. Such findings contribute to a growing body of evidence that nutritional science plays a pivotal role in extending human lifespans and improving overall health quality. Understanding the biochemical underpinnings that link nutrition to longevity is crucial in optimizing dietary patterns for extended health. Recent studies have highlighted the significance of epigenetic mechanisms, where dietary choices influence gene expression without altering the underlying DNA sequence. These epigenetic modifications can result from micronutrient availability, dietary fats, and other bioactive compounds found in food, each contributing to cellular repair and inflammation regulation. The impact of gut microbiota on longevity is an emerging frontier; specific dietary fibers promote a diverse and healthy gut microbiome, which has been correlated with improved metabolic health and reduced inflammation markers. The interconnectedness of dietary components and biological aging, as portrayed in, underlines the potential for tailored nutritional interventions to mitigate age-related decline. This complex relationship emphasizes that a holistic approach, integrating diverse nutritional elements, may significantly enhance longevity prospects. The cultural dimensions of dietary practices also play a profound role in the pursuit of longevity. As different societies adopt various nutritional philosophies aimed at promoting health and longevity, understanding these cultural values can yield insights into sustainable practices. The traditional Blue Zone diets showcase how lifestyle choices— ranging from plant-based diets to community engagement—are harmonized to achieve longevity. These findings underline the fundamental role of nutrition not just as a biochemical intervention but as part of a broader lifestyle framework. The intersection of nutrition with social determinants of health bolsters the argument for a multifaceted approach to lifespan extension, reinforcing the notion that simply prolonging life is insufficient. Instead, it is vital to cultivate an environment where quality of life remains a priority, as suggested in the visual systems of interconnected health determinants shown in. Thus, it becomes evident that fostering a balanced nutritional landscape is essential in navigating the complexities of future longevity initiatives.

Role of Diet in Aging

Diet plays a pivotal role in influencing the aging process, serving as a key contributor to both longevity and the quality of life in later years. Research has shown that specific dietary patterns can dramatically impact the biological mechanisms underlying aging. Diets rich in whole, unprocessed foods, such as those found in the Mediterranean dietary pattern, have been associated with reduced inflammation and lower incidences of age-related diseases. The connection between nutrition and chronic illnesses, including heart disease, diabetes, and even cognitive decline, highlights the necessity of adopting dietary habits that enhance health span rather than merely lifespan. As stated in studies on dietary impacts, Diet is a critical component of healthy aging, and it's not just about what you eat, but also what you don't eat, reinforcing the importance of mindful consumption practices in mitigating the adverse effects of aging. Incorporating this understanding into public health policies could offer strategic pathways to improve population health as life expectancy expands. A caloric restriction strategy has garnered attention in recent years, particularly due to its remarkable effects on extending lifespan in various animal models. This approach, which emphasizes a significant reduction in daily caloric intake without sacrificing nutritional quality, has the potential to activate critical cellular pathways that promote longevity. Research suggests that living with restricted caloric intake minimizes instances of metabolic disorders and enhances the body's regenerative capabilities. As scientists delve deeper into the impacts of caloric restriction, they discover that this dietary pattern may enhance the efficiency of cellular repair mechanisms, translating to healthier aging and potentially curbing the onset of age-related diseases. The endorsement of caloric restriction as a lifestyle modification aligns with emerging discussions around dietary interventions as tools in longevity research. Such findings not only offer individual benefits but also imply broader implications for health care systems grappling with aging populations. The emerging concept of nutrition's interplay with biological aging emphasizes the need for a more holistic view of diet. Studies have demonstrated that the gut-brain axis plays a crucial role in mediating the relationship between dietary choices and aging. Changes in microbiota composition, influenced by dietary habits, can impact inflammation, metabolic regulation, and even mental health. As the body ages, the microbiome undergoes significant changes, which can exacerbate health challenges if not properly managed through diet. Hence, addressing dietary intake in older adults may not only improve gut health but also enhance overall well-being. As our understanding of these complex relationships deepens, there is a pressing need for more personalized dietary interventions tailored to individual health profiles. Such advancements in nutritional science could serve as vital components of the broader frameworks aimed at promoting healthy longevity, ultimately shaping the discourse around sustainable living into old age.

Caloric Restriction and Its Effects

In recent years, research has increasingly focused on the effects of caloric restriction on longevity. This approach posits that reducing caloric intake without malnutrition can trigger a cascade of biological responses that enhance lifespan and health span.

Studies across various model organisms, including yeast and rodents, have shown promising results, suggesting that caloric restriction activates key cellular pathways related to aging. Reductions in calorie intake appear to initiate mechanisms involving the insulin/IGF-1 signaling pathway, which plays a critical role in growth and metabolism. As articulated in the literature, *"Caloric restriction has been shown to extend lifespan in various animal models, including yeast, worms, flies, and rodents." (David B. Allison and others)*. This evidence suggests that further exploration of caloric restriction could provide pivotal insights into not only improving the quantity of life but also maintaining the quality of life—a crucial consideration for the pursuit of extended longevity. The biochemical effects of caloric restriction also shed light on potential therapeutic applications for age-related diseases. Researchers have observed that caloric restriction may enhance autophagy, a process whereby cells effectively recycle damaged components. This cellular cleanup could play a vital role in mitigating conditions commonly associated with aging, such as neurodegenerative diseases and metabolic disorders. Studies indicate that caloric restriction can positively influence inflammatory responses, which are often exacerbated in older populations. As the scientific community delves into the intricacies of these mechanisms, findings suggest that understanding how caloric restriction alters metabolic pathways may yield new avenues for interventions in human health. Consequently, a deeper investigation into the interplay between caloric intake and disease prevention could be instrumental in addressing societal challenges associated with longevity. While the potential benefits of caloric restriction are promising, they must be weighed against practical considerations for implementation in human populations. Adherence to caloric restriction as a long-term health strategy often raises questions regarding individual variability, sustainability, and social implications. The psychological challenges of significantly altering dietary patterns, especially in cultures where abundance is celebrated, cannot be overlooked. Additionally, the risk of nutrient deficiencies and the importance of balanced intake underscore the need for guided approaches to caloric restriction. Future research must not only focus on the biological underpinnings of caloric restriction but also consider behavioral and societal factors that influence dietary choices. By doing so, the scientific community can formulate comprehensive strategies that equip individuals to navigate the complexities of dietary changes in the context of extended life expectancy. Integrating findings from studies like those depicted in will enhance our understanding of caloric restrictions multifaceted effects on health and longevity, ultimately contributing to a more nuanced discourse on the subject.

Study	Caloric Restriction (%)	Average Lifespan Increase (%)	Species
University of Texas (2018)	30	25	Rhesus Monkeys
National Institute on Aging (2020)	20	15	Lab Mice
Buck Institute for Research on Aging (2019)	40	50	Yeast
University of Southern California (2021)	30	20	Fruit Flies
Harvard Medical School (2017)	25	30	Roundworms

Caloric Restriction Studies and Life Expectancy

Supplements and Longevity

Modern society has increasingly gravitated toward the use of dietary supplements as a means to promote health and longevity. This reflects a growing awareness of the interplay between lifestyle choices and the aging process. Supplements, ranging from essential vitamins to specialized compounds like antioxidants and omega-3 fatty acids, are often marketed with claims that they can significantly enhance physical health and extend life expectancy. Critical evaluation reveals that while some research supports the benefits of specific supplements, many health claims lack sufficient evidence regarding their effectiveness. The question remains whether these products truly contribute to longevity or if they merely represent a modern panacea amidst widespread health anxieties. As noted, the use of dietary supplements is a common practice among individuals seeking to enhance their health and longevity, yet it is paramount to approach these with a critical and evidence-based mindset, ensuring that supplementation complements rather than substitutes a wholesome diet and healthy lifestyle choices. A closer examination of the prevailing attitudes toward supplements highlights both potential benefits and pitfalls in the quest for longevity. Some studies suggest that certain supplements may positively impact health markers that are indirectly associated with aging, such as cardiovascular health and cognitive function. The efficacy of these supplements often varies widely among individuals, influenced by factors such as genetics, existing health conditions, and overall dietary patterns. Additionally, the unregulated nature of the supplement industry poses risks, as products may not always contain the advertised ingredients or dosages. Thus, while some individuals may experience benefits, it is crucial to approach supplementation as an adjunct to, rather than a replacement for, established health practices. Public health messages should emphasize that, nutritional supplements can play a role in supporting overall health, but they should not replace a balanced diet, encouraging a well-rounded approach to health that prioritizes whole foods and lifestyle modifications. The exploration of supplements and their relationship to longevity directs attention to the broader implications of nutrition in the aging process. As emerging research reinforces the significance of nutrient-rich diets in promoting longevity, the conversation shifts toward how these practices can be integrated into daily life. Communities that prioritize healthy eating patterns—such as those emphasized in the Mediterranean diet—often demonstrate lower rates of age-related diseases and improved quality of life in older adults. This emphasizes a crucial consideration in future discussions on longevity: that the foundations of health should lie within accessible, whole-food options rather than solely in supplement use. Integrating this perspective can enable individuals to make informed dietary choices that foster lasting well-being, ultimately shaping a societal environment that supports a healthier, longer life. Dependence on supplements without a harmonious relationship with proper nutrition may detract from achieving true longevity goals.

VIII. MENTAL HEALTH AND LONGEVITY

The intricate interplay between mental well-being and longevity has garnered increasing attention in contemporary research, illuminating a crucial yet often overlooked aspect of aging. As individuals navigate the complexities of modern life, factors such as stress, anxiety, and depression significantly impact their overall health. Studies have shown that chronic stress can lead to physiological changes that negatively affect the immune system, thereby increasing susceptibility to various diseases. When mental health deteriorates, it can manifest physically, presenting challenges to maintaining a high quality of life in old age. Consequently, a holistic approach that promotes mental resilience alongside physical health emerges as a fundamental aspect of longevity research. Understanding that mental health is just as important as physical health underscores the necessity of addressing both realms to foster an environment conducive to living well throughout an extended lifespan *"Mental health is just as important as physical health, and it's essential to address both to achieve overall well-being and longevity." (Dr. Laura L. Carstensen).* Delving deeper, the role of social connections in promoting mental and emotional health provides another layer of understanding in the quest for longevity. Research indicates that strong relationships and social engagement can mitigate feelings of loneliness and depression, significantly influencing an individual's life expectancy. The importance of community, as described in various studies on aging, highlights that individuals who maintain active social lives tend to display better cognitive function and emotional regulation. This suggests a multi-faceted relationship where supportive social networks not only enhance mental health but also provide the emotional scaffolding necessary for navigating the challenges of aging. As families and societies evolve in their approach to longevity, a shift towards valuing emotional well-being as a protective factor for physical health could emerge as a pivotal element in both personal and public health strategies. Understanding the impact of modern lifestyle choices on mental health offers critical insights into strategies for enhancing longevity. Factors such as diet, exercise, and sleep patterns are intricately linked to mental well-being and, consequently, longevity. Engaging in regular physical activity has been shown to reduce stress, improve mood, and even sharpen cognitive function. Additionally, dietary choices that prioritize nutritional balance can affect mental health and resilience. Advancements in the field of nutrition and mental health reveal a clear connection between what we consume and our psychological state, emphasizing the significance of dietary interventions in promoting longevity. As the quest for a longer lifespan continues, integrating mental health strategies alongside traditional healthcare practices will become increasingly essential, positioning mental wellness as a cornerstone in the broader narrative of aging and living well.

Psychological Well-being in Old Age

Psychological well-being in old age is intricately linked to several factors, most notably ones social network and engagement levels. As individuals age, the shift often leads to the loss of social connections through retirement, the passing of friends, or health-related mobility restrictions. This loss can trigger feelings of isolation and despair, detrimentally impacting mental health.

Conversely, maintaining rich social interactions has been shown to bolster psychological resilience. Indeed, studies suggest that social engagement plays a pivotal role in successful aging. Healthy relationships promote emotional support, shared experiences, and a sense of belonging, which are crucial for anyone navigating the complexities of old age. These findings underscore the necessity of proactive community-building initiatives aimed at fostering social ties among seniors, enhancing their overall quality of life and sense of purpose *"Older adults who maintain a sense of purpose and meaning in life tend to have better psychological well-being." (Laura L. Carstensen)*. Thus, a focus on social engagement is paramount in strategies aimed at promoting psychological well-being in older adults. The concept of purpose and meaning in life cannot be underestimated when discussing psychological well-being during aging. Individuals who perceive a sense of purpose tend to engage more actively with life, exhibiting higher levels of contentment and lower incidences of depression. The search for meaning often reinforces personal identity, offering older adults a framework through which they can evaluate their experiences and navigate challenges associated with aging. Engaging in post-retirement projects, volunteering, or nurturing family relationships can provide a renewed sense of purpose. As such, psychological theories and practices that encourage a purposeful lifestyle should be integral to geriatric care. Older adults who maintain a sense of purpose and meaning in life tend to have better psychological well-being, as evidenced by a plethora of research finding significant correlations between purpose and emotional resilience in late life. Establishing environments conducive to fostering these meaningful engagements can profoundly enhance well-being and satisfaction. A multifaceted approach to psychological well-being in older adults must also consider the biological factors intertwined with mental health. Scientific advancements in understanding aging biomarkers penetrate deeply into how psychological well-being is perceived and maintained. Variations in genetic factors can influence not just the onset of age-related diseases but also the psychological resilience of older adults. Emerging fields like epigenetics are revealing how lifestyle choices—such as diet and exercise—interact with these genetic predispositions to shape psychological outcomes. This confluence of biological, social, and psychological factors presents an opportunity for more holistic elder care. By adopting an integrative view that spans biological age markers and psychological factors, caregivers can tailor interventions that address the unique needs of the elderly, thereby optimizing their emotional health and enhancing their overall quality of life as they navigate the challenges of prolonged longevity. This comprehensive approach holds the key to unlocking better mental health and satisfaction in old age.

Cognitive Decline and Prevention

Expanding our understanding of cognitive decline requires a multifaceted approach that encompasses not only biological factors but also lifestyle influences. Aging is often accompanied by a gradual decline in cognitive function, leading to concerns about dementia and other cognitive disorders. As research indicates, preventive strategies are essential for mitigating these effects. Engaging in regular physical activity, maintaining a balanced diet, and fostering social connections have all been linked to improved cognitive health. In fact, one prominent study highlights that lifestyle interventions, including physical activity, cognitive training, and social engagement, can have a positive impact on cognitive health in older adults. *"Cognitive decline is a complex and multifactorial process, influenced by a combination of genetic, environmental, and lifestyle factors. Preventive strategies, such as regular physical activity, a balanced diet, social engagement, and cognitive stimulation, have been shown to reduce the risk of cognitive decline and dementia."* (Laura Fratiglioni). Such findings point toward a holistic model of health, wherein the protection of cognitive function is viewed as a collective effort involving individual actions and community resources. This model not only addresses symptoms but also enables proactive management of cognitive health as life expectancy extends. Additionally, the integration of modern technologies and scientific advances plays a crucial role in the prevention of cognitive decline. With growing evidence supporting the efficacy of personalized medicine, interventions tailored to individual genetic and environmental profiles are becoming more prevalent. This personalized approach allows for targeted strategies that consider specific risk factors for cognitive impairment. Emerging technologies such as artificial intelligence are being utilized to analyze large datasets, generating insights that can be applied to design interventions that delay cognitive decline. The elucidation of biological aging mechanisms, as illustrated in various studies, emphasizes the need for innovative solutions that address the causes of cognitive dysfunction at their roots. By leveraging these advancements in biology and technology, we can create frameworks that proactively promote cognitive resilience as we navigate the challenges of increased longevity. The implications of cognitive decline extend beyond the individual, influencing familial and societal structures. As life expectancy rises, communities must adapt to the increasing demands of an aging population. This shift includes fostering environments conducive to mental wellness and social interaction, which are essential for preventing isolation and cognitive deterioration. Policymakers and health organizations have begun to recognize the interdependence of cognitive health and overall societal wellbeing, encouraging initiatives that facilitate healthy aging. The focus on creating supportive communities aligns with the notion that cognitive decline is a complex and multifactorial process, influenced by a combination of genetic, environmental, and lifestyle factors. This broader perspective not only prepares us for the societal challenges of extended lifespans but also reinforces the importance of community engagement in safeguarding cognitive health, ultimately ensuring a higher quality of life as we approach the future of longevity.

Social Connections and Longevity

In examining the intricate relationship between social connections and longevity, it becomes evident that human interaction plays a pivotal role in shaping health outcomes across the lifespan. The profound impact of strong social ties can be observed in various studies that indicate individuals with robust social networks are more likely to enjoy a longer life. A critical aspect of this phenomenon lies in how social relationships contribute to improved mental well-being and physical health. Engaging in regular interactions reduces stress, promotes emotional support, and encourages healthier lifestyles. Friends and family often motivate one another to maintain fitness or adhere to medical regimens, significantly affecting ones overall health trajectory. Research highlights that *"Social relationships, or the relative lack thereof, constitute a major risk factor for health— rivaling the effect of well-established health risk factors such as smoking, blood pressure, and lipid levels."* (Holt-Lunstad, Julianne). This compelling evidence underscores the importance of nurturing social bonds not only for immediate emotional satisfaction but also for enhancing longevity. Delving deeper into the mechanisms by which social connections influence longevity, it is essential to consider the biological and psychological pathways involved. Social interactions can trigger positive physiological responses, such as the release of hormones that bolster resilience against stress and inflammation. Additionally, supportive relationships foster a sense of purpose and belonging, which are crucial for mental health. The implications of these findings challenge individuals to prioritize social engagement as a vital component of their wellness routine. Notably, the protective effects of social ties have been linked to decreased instances of chronic illness and higher rates of recovery. Studies illustrate that people with stronger social relationships had a 50% increased likelihood of survival over the study period, emphasizing the crucial role of community and connectedness in long-term health. Understanding these dynamics paves the way for public health interventions that integrate social support systems into health promotion strategies. The implications of fostering social connections extend beyond individual health, reaching into the broader societal landscape as we consider the future of longevity. As advancements in biotechnology and healthcare allow for increased life expectancy, the concept of societal engagement becomes increasingly significant. An aging population that is socially active not only experiences improved health outcomes but also contributes to a vibrant community, enriching societal dynamics and collaboration. Conversely, isolation can lead to increased healthcare burdens and diminished quality of life, complicating the ethical landscape surrounding life extension. As we curate environments that promote companionship and mutual support, the challenge lies in translating these findings into actionable policies that prioritize social infrastructure alongside health innovations. The importance of fostering social interactions in this context emphasizes that longevity isn't just about living longer but living well, advocating for a holistic approach that intertwines physical health with deep-rooted social connections.

Year	Study	Findings
2020	Harvard Study of Adult Development	Strong social connections were linked to a 50% increased chance of survival
2021	National Institute on Aging	Having few social connections can shorten lifespan by up to 15 years
2022	American Journal of Epidemiology	Loneliness increases the risk of premature death by 26%
2023	University of Michigan	Social isolation in older adults is associated with a 29% increased risk of mortality
2023	Pew Research Center	Individuals with strong social networks report higher levels of happiness and lower physical decline

Social Connections and Longevity Data

IX. ECONOMIC IMPLICATIONS OF EXTENDED LIFESPAN

The potential economic implications accompanying an extended lifespan are vast and complex. As advancements in healthcare and technology improve life expectancy, the dynamics of the labor market will inevitably shift. Older individuals may opt to remain in the workforce longer, capitalizing on their accumulated experience and skills. This prolonged engagement presents opportunities for economic growth, as a more seasoned and knowledgeable workforce could enhance productivity and foster innovation within various sectors. This shift could also entail increased competition for job opportunities among younger workers, potentially leading to tensions in the labor market. A critical examination of these dynamics must address not only the benefits of a longer-lived population contributing to economic activity but also the associated challenges, such as the need for retraining programs tailored to the evolving roles of older employees. Such challenges underscore the intricate balance between leveraging longevity as an economic asset while mitigating potential workforce disparities. The increasing demand for healthcare services and resources among a growing elderly population poses significant economic challenges. With longer lifespans come heightened risks of chronic diseases and health-related issues that demand sustained medical attention. Social security systems and pension plans may strain under the weight of a demographic increasingly skewed towards older age groups. As stated in a recent analysis, the social security systems, pension funds, and healthcare resources face significant strains due to this shift in population demographics *"The economic implications of extended lifespan are multifaceted and far-reaching. On one hand, a longer-lived population could contribute to increased economic productivity and innovation. On the other hand, it could also lead to significant strains on social security systems, pension funds, and healthcare resources." (David A. Sinclair).* Policymakers must therefore critically assess current welfare structures and explore innovative financial solutions to ensure sustainability. The projected rise in healthcare expenditure necessitates a reevaluation of healthcare delivery models, prioritizing preventative care and efficient resource allocation to maintain quality of life while curbing costs. Planning for these economic ramifications will be essential in adapting to the realities of extended longevity. An extended lifespan invites a profound rethinking of societal priorities and intergenerational dynamics. The traditional model of life stages—education, work, and retirement—may no longer fit a reality of living well into ones 150s. As individuals extend their productive years, questions surrounding retirement age, social contributions, and familial roles become pressing. Individuals who might have retired in their sixties may find themselves engaged in careers or community service well into their later years. This shift could positively influence family structures by nurturing multigenerational interactions, where wisdom and skills are shared among age groups. It also necessitates a redesign of economic systems to accommodate changes in family dynamics and caregiving responsibilities. Policies that promote life-long learning and flexibility in work arrangements would be integral to ensuring that society can adapt smoothly to these changes while enabling individuals to live fulfilling lives at all stages. By embedding this proactive approach within societal planning, we can better prepare for the economic implications of living longer, healthier lives.

Year	Global Life Expectancy (Years)	Average Retirement Age (Years)	Projected Health Care Costs per Senior ($)
2020	72.6	65	15,000
2025	73.4	65	17,000
2030	74.5	66	20,000
2035	75.6	67	23,000
2040	76.5	68	26,000

Economic Implications of Extended Lifespan

Impact on Healthcare Systems

In the continuously evolving landscape of healthcare, the implications of extending life expectancy significantly reshape the contours of health systems. As technological innovations in biomedicine allow for people to live longer, our current healthcare infrastructure may find itself overwhelmed if proactive measures are not taken. The multifaceted approach to health, as shown in, emphasizes crucial areas like molecular design and mental health analysis, which will inform how healthcare providers respond to the needs of an aging population. This implies that healthcare systems must not only expand their capacity to deliver complex services but also enhance their focus on preventative care and integrated treatments that address the complexities of age-related conditions. The shift from reactive to proactive care would require systemic changes, including workforce training, interdisciplinary collaboration, and technological adaptations that better align with this new understanding of longevity. The societal implications of increased life expectancy challenge not only healthcare delivery but also economic structures and social services. As indicated in, various dietary approaches can influence aging and health outcomes, suggesting that wellness-oriented policies could be more broadly integrated into healthcare systems. Governments might need to reallocate budgets and resources toward preventive strategies that promote healthier lifestyles, thereby reducing the long-term costs associated with chronic diseases common in aging populations. As populations age, there is likely to be a greater emphasis on mental health and well-being, necessitating healthcare models that prioritize holistic approaches. The integration of data from multiple disciplines and methodologies, as depicted in, will be instrumental in shaping policies that effectively respond to this demographic shift by prioritizing preventive care over illness management. The ethical considerations surrounding increased longevity cannot be overlooked, as they play a critical role in shaping healthcare systems of the future. The images illustrating comprehensive biological mechanisms, like those in, underscore the ethical dilemmas associated with advancing medical technologies, such as genetic editing and regenerative therapies. While these advancements may extend life expectancy, they also pose questions of equity, access, and the moral implications of extending life at the expense of quality of life. Many cultures grapple with their perceptions of aging, as highlighted in the overall context of these images. Healthcare policymakers need to consider the varied reactions from society and how these perspectives affect acceptance and integration of longevity-related innovations. Fostering a healthcare system that can adapt and thrive in the context of increased longevity will demand not only scientific and technical advancements but a nuanced understanding of ethical frameworks and societal values.

Workforce Dynamics and Retirement

The increasing longevity of individuals raises complex challenges for workforce dynamics, particularly around the concepts of work and retirement. As people live longer, traditional paradigms regarding retirement age and workforce participation need reevaluation. With the potential for extended lifespans, the standard retirement age of 65 may soon become obsolete, demanding a shift toward more flexible work arrangements. More companies are beginning to recognize that experienced workers can bring invaluable skills and institutional knowledge, making it essential to create an environment where older employees can thrive. As outlined in *"As people live longer, the traditional retirement age will need to be reevaluated to accommodate a longer and healthier workforce." (Laura L. Carstensen)*, the traditional retirement age will need to be reevaluated to accommodate a longer and healthier workforce. To effectively harness the capabilities of older workers, organizations must adopt strategies that blend intergenerational collaboration and lifelong learning opportunities, ensuring that the workforce remains dynamic and adaptable in the face of demographic changes. The implication of extended lifespans on workforce participation extends beyond just the retirement age; it requires a cultural shift in how we perceive aging in the workplace. More than simply enabling older employees to remain in their roles, organizations must cultivate inclusive environments that celebrate diverse age cohorts. Research has shown that combining insights from younger generations with the expertise of seasoned professionals leads to enhanced problem-solving and innovation. Health and wellness programs tailored to older employees could also prolong their work-life, increasing both productivity and job satisfaction. The transition to a multi-generational workforce raises important questions about training and mentorship, necessitating new frameworks for knowledge transfer and skill development. Such initiatives must be firmly rooted in the understanding that healthy aging is a societal goal, effectively removing age-related stigmas and enabling a collective maturation of the workforce. The redefinition of retirement will be crucial in addressing the psychological and financial aspects of a longer life. For many, the traditional model of retirement represents the culmination of a career, a time of relaxation and travel. As longevity becomes a norm, a more fluid approach to career breaks and ongoing professional engagement may emerge instead. Encouraging phased retirement, where older workers gradually reduce their hours while mentoring younger colleagues, could provide an effective transition. This dual approach not only aids in knowledge transmission but also addresses the potential financial burdens that come with living longer lives. Reinventing retirement as a period of exploration rather than withdrawal aligns with shifting societal values towards continuous learning and self-fulfillment. As we consider the future challenges of longevity, it is imperative to establish a framework that supports healthy aging while fostering a vibrant, engaged workforce.

Year	Over 65 in Workforce (%)	Average Retirement Age	Life Expectancy Years
2020	19.3	66	78.8
2021	19.5	66	79.1
2022	19.8	66.1	79.3
2023	20	66.3	79.5
2024	20.5	66.5	79.8

Workforce Dynamics and Retirement Data

Economic Opportunities in Longevity Industries

As advancements in biotechnology and regenerative medicine continue to unfold, an array of economic opportunities are arising within the longevity industry. The exploration into cellular aging processes and genetic interventions presents substantial potential for market growth, attracting significant investments from venture capital and corporate entities. This burgeoning sector not only promises new therapeutic modalities that could revolutionize healthcare but also offers a fertile ground for innovation in related fields such as pharmaceuticals, diagnostics, and wearable health technology. Companies that successfully leverage these advances are likely to play pivotal roles in creating products and services tailored to enhance the health and longevity of aging populations. Indeed, the longevity industry is positioned to transform traditional healthcare paradigms, extending beyond mere disease treatment to encompass proactive health management strategies and preventive measures. Such a shift is crucial for addressing the myriad health challenges associated with an aging demographic, facilitating both individual well-being and broader economic sustainability. The intersection of digital technology and longevity research underscores another layer of economic opportunity. As digital health tools become integrated into daily life, startups focused on data analytics, artificial intelligence, and machine learning are emerging, aiming to personalize and optimize longevity-related healthcare services. The growth of telemedicine and decentralized clinical trials leads to increased accessibility and efficiency in health interventions, responding to the needs of both individuals and healthcare providers. As noted, *"The economic opportunities in the longevity sector are vast and multifaceted. From pharmaceuticals and biotechnology to healthcare services and technology, the potential for innovation and investment is significant. As people live longer, healthier lives, new markets and industries will emerge to meet their needs."* (Andrew J. Scott), encompassing a variety of market segments, including wellness products, nutraceuticals, and lifestyle programs that cater to the aging population. This multifaceted approach to health not only drives innovation but also spurs job creation across diverse sectors, reinforcing the narrative of longevity as a catalyst for economic growth. Addressing the complex ethical, social, and economic challenges posed by longevity sciences is imperative for the industry's sustainable development. As the potential for significantly extended lifespans becomes more viable, societal implications—including employment patterns, healthcare costs, and resource allocation—must be examined. The prospect of an aging population requires a reimagining of workforce dynamics; older individuals may increasingly participate in the workforce, necessitating changes in policies concerning retirement, training, and health benefits. Businesses that proactively adapt to these shifts, by investing in continuous learning and health-centric programs, will find themselves at a distinct advantage. The ability to create products that enhance quality of life while addressing the unique needs of older adults not only fulfills a growing demand but also contributes to fostering societal resilience in the face of demographic change. This holistic approach outlines a pathway for economic expansion while ensuring that advances in longevity translate into tangible benefits for individuals and society alike.

Year	Market Size (Billion USD)	Expected Growth Rate (%)
2020	121	7.5
2021	130	8.0
2022	139	8.5
2023	150	9.0
2024 (Projected)	162	9.5
2025 (Projected)	175	10.0

Economic Opportunities in Longevity Industries

X. ETHICAL DILEMMAS OF LONGEVITY

Ethical dilemmas surrounding longevity extend into the realm of resource allocation, posing fundamental questions about societal priorities. The prospect of extending human life significantly, perhaps into the realm of 150 years, demands a reevaluation of how we distribute healthcare resources. As individuals age, their medical needs typically increase, leading to a potential strain on healthcare systems that are already grappling with inefficiencies and growing patient populations. These challenges highlight the urgent need for equitable access to medical advancements among diverse socio-economic groups. The ramifications of prolonged life expectancy could exacerbate existing disparities, as individuals from underprivileged backgrounds may not receive the same level of care or access to life-extending treatments. As noted in the dialogue on longevity, the pursuit of longevity raises complex ethical questions about the distribution of resources, emphasizing the critical need to address social justice within the discourse on ethical longevity *"As people live longer, there will be increased pressure on healthcare systems, pension funds, and other social services, which can lead to ethical dilemmas about how to allocate resources." (Dr. Aubrey de Grey)*. Addressing these disparities is essential for ensuring that advancements in life extension foster overall societal well-being rather than reinforce inequity. The implications of extended lifespan extend beyond individual health; they reverberate throughout societal structures and family dynamics. As people live longer, traditional definitions of family, community, and labor may shift radically. The extended presence of elderly family members could alter built-in support systems, placing increased emotional and financial burdens on younger generations. Prolonged working life may raise challenges related to career progression and the job market, potentially resulting in age-related discrimination. Ethical considerations need to confront the question of whether society is prepared to accommodate an aging population in terms of employment opportunities, social services, and familial responsibilities. As society grapples with these dynamics, the prospect of longevity holds the risk that increased pressure on healthcare systems, pension funds, and other social services can lead to ethical dilemmas, thereby necessitating comprehensive policy adaptations to navigate the implications of this demographic shift. The potential for significant advancements in biotechnology and regenerative medicine raises pressing ethical questions regarding consent and the concept of natural life spans. As scientists explore genetic editing and other modalities to enhance life quality and extend lifespan, the line between natural aging processes and artificially prolonged life becomes blurred. This raises questions about who should have access to these technologies and the ethical implications of their use. The risk exists that such resources may only be available to wealthier individuals or nations, exacerbating existing inequalities. This newfound capability might prompt dilemmas concerning the societal worth of aging, with implications for how we perceive the elderly in various cultures. To navigate these challenges, it is vital to promote inclusive dialogue that encourages ethical standards in the development and application of life-extending technologies. The conversation around longevity cannot be limited to mere lifespan extension but must encompass a broader understanding of quality of life and equitable access to innovations that could fundamentally transform human existence.

Equity in Access to Longevity Technologies

The emergence of advanced longevity technologies, while promising increased lifespan and better health outcomes, raises profound ethical considerations regarding equitable access. As regenerative medicine, genetic editing, and other innovations evolve, disparities in socioeconomic status could dictate who benefits from these advancements. Those in lower-income brackets may find themselves excluded from life-extending treatments due to high costs or lack of availability. This scenario could reinforce existing health inequities, leading to a society where only a privileged few enjoy the fruits of prolonged life. The complexity of these technologies further complicates the situation, as an understanding of their implications and access to education about them will vary widely across different communities. Highlighting these disparities, researchers must emphasize that the equitable distribution of longevity technologies is crucial for ensuring that the benefits of extended lifespan are not limited to a privileged few but are accessible to all segments of society *"The equitable distribution of longevity technologies is crucial for ensuring that the benefits of extended lifespan are not limited to a privileged few, but are accessible to all segments of society." (Dr. Laura L. Carstensen)*. This awareness is necessary to foster a society that promotes longevity for all individuals, irrespective of their background. Diverse community perspectives will play a crucial role in shaping equitable access to longevity technologies. Understanding the cultural, social, and economic context of different populations is essential in navigating potential barriers. Initiatives focusing on public education and community engagement can help demystify longevity technologies and gather data on the needs and preferences of underrepresented groups. A grassroots approach involving local stakeholders can facilitate more inclusive dialogue about the implementation and accessibility of these technologies. Collaboration between government, healthcare providers, private industry, and communities can lead to innovative solutions that promote equity in health outcomes. By investing in healthcare infrastructure and prioritizing accessible education, these partnerships can help alleviate the gap between those who can afford cutting-edge longevity treatments and those who cannot. Addressing these disparities will ensure that advancements in longevity technologies benefit the broader society rather than deepen existing inequalities. Tackling the issue of equity in access to longevity technologies will demand a multifaceted strategy that incorporates policy reform, ethical frameworks, and inclusion strategies. Governments and policymakers must legislate to ensure equitable distribution of resources and protections against discrimination in healthcare access. Without such active measures, the advancement of longevity technologies risks perpetuating health disparities, creating a society divided not only by wealth but also by lifespan. The ethical dimensions of access must be included in discussions about developing these technologies. Key players in the field, including researchers, clinicians, and bioethicists, must collaborate to create guidelines that prioritize fairness in healthcare access. The image depicting the relationships among various health-determinant factors underscores the need for synergy between individual, community, and population-level health strategies. It reflects how grassroots reform can act as a catalyst for sustainable changes that promote equality in longevity technologies. Ensuring broad availability of these advancements will be instrumental in shaping a future where health equity contributes to an improved quality of life for all, irrespective of their socioeconomic status.

Moral Implications of Life Extension

The potential for extended lifespans presents a range of ethical dilemmas that challenge our moral frameworks. As advancements in biotechnology and regenerative medicine close the gap between possibility and reality, society must grapple with questions that probe the very essence of existence. Among these questions, the concern about exacerbating existing social inequalities arises prominently. If life extension technologies remain accessible primarily to the wealthy, the divide between socioeconomic classes could deepen. Those without access may experience a reduced quality of life due to health disparities, feeding into a cycle of privilege and disadvantage. Such discrepancies arise from our current healthcare systems, which often reflect broader societal inequalities. To sustain a just society, it is imperative to explore equitable access to these life-extending technologies, thereby ensuring that every individual has a fair chance to benefit from advancements in longevity without being marginalized by socioeconomic barriers. provides a visual representation of this multifaceted issue by exploring the potential benefits across various demographics. The implications of life extension extend beyond individual access and social equity; they also encompass profound moral considerations regarding resource allocation and environmental sustainability. An aging population living significantly longer could place immense pressure on already strained resources, such as healthcare systems, social services, and the environment. The prospect of overpopulation driven by increased longevity raises questions about the planets ability to sustain its inhabitants. As noted in the discourse surrounding this issue, extending human lifespan without addressing ecological consequences could lead to significant social and environmental challenges. Consequently, decision-makers must grapple with the ethical responsibility of ensuring sustainable solutions alongside the pursuit of longevity. This calls for interdisciplinary approaches that incorporate ethical frameworks and scientific understanding, allowing society to innovate responsibly. A systems-level analysis of aging, as illustrated in, underscores the interconnectedness of health, ecological stability, and resource distribution, highlighting the need for comprehensive strategies. The moral implications of life extension reveal an intricate web of considerations that demands our attention. While extending human life presents opportunities for individuals to contribute meaningfully to society, it also brings forth ethical challenges regarding equity, resource distribution, and environmental sustainability. The balancing act of promoting longevity while safeguarding the integrity of ecosystems and social contracts is a monumental task. It is crucial to approach this frontier with a sense of collective responsibility to ensure that advancements in life extension serve the greater good, rather than perpetuating existing inequities. As we contemplate our future, we must heed the warning that, as one observer noted, would life extension exacerbate existing social and economic inequalities, or would it provide new opportunities for personal and societal growth?. *"The prospect of significantly extending human lifespan raises a host of ethical questions. Would life extension exacerbate existing social and economic inequalities, or would it provide new opportunities for personal and societal growth?" (Leonard Hayflick).* This inquiry should shape ongoing dialogues about the direction humanity takes in the pursuit of longevity, pushing us to consider the profound social contract at stake. As depicted in, understanding the determinants of health becomes a pivotal aspect of shaping policies and practices related to life extension.

The Value of Life and Death

Life's inherent value is often contemplated through the lens of mortality, prompting questions about the significance of our experiences and the legacy we leave behind. The pursuit of extending life raises philosophical inquiries regarding what it means to live meaningfully, especially in a world where technological advancements promise greater longevity. As we evaluate the implications of living to 150 years, it is essential to consider not only the biological aspects of aging but also the broader context of human existence. This includes the quality of life, the relationships we foster, and the accomplishments we strive for. The intricate interplay between life and death shapes our behaviors, motivations, and aspirations, ultimately crafting a narrative where death acts as a catalyst for valuing our time on earth. This theme resonates through emerging discussions in fields such as reinforcement learning and health analysis, as illustrated in, where the intricate connections between mental health and biological age highlight the importance of depth in understanding the human experience. The societal consequences of extended lifespans cannot be ignored, as they prompt a reevaluation of how we perceive death and the end of life. A longer life may lead to richer experiences and opportunities; however, it also poses complex ethical dilemmas concerning resource allocation, healthcare, and the economic impacts of an aging population. This multifaceted discourse is critical when considering whether society is prepared for such a drastic change in life expectancy. A notable aspect of this debate revolves around the maxim that *"The extension of human lifespan is a complex issue that involves not just the biological and medical aspects, but also ethical, social, and economic considerations." (Dr. David A. Sinclair)*. Such insights force us to confront the moral implications of longevity technologies while grappling with the potential for increasing disparities in health access and outcomes. The tension between enhanced longevity and the potential devaluation of life's perennial cycles calls for a careful consideration of societal values, particularly as illustrated in the frameworks of aging progression in. Examining the value of life and death within the context of cultural perspectives offers additional depth to this discussion. Different societies hold varying views on aging, death, and the profound meaning often derived from these experiences. In some cultures, death is celebrated as a natural transition, while others perceive it as a significant loss that necessitates mourning. This multifaceted viewpoint shapes individuals understandings of their roles in familial and communal contexts, influencing how longevity is perceived and valued. The embrace of life-affirming practices can provide a counterpoint to the fears surrounding death, suggesting that a shift in our collective mindset could pave the way for a healthier relationship with aging. Images that illustrate the integration of multi-omics approaches to health analysis, like those in, underpin the notion that understanding aging can lead to improved quality of life, thereby addressing the essential question of whether we are ready to embrace a future where life extends significantly.

XI. SOCIAL DYNAMICS OF AN AGING POPULATION

The interactions of an aging population within society are multifaceted, encompassing shifts in familial roles and community engagements. As demographics transition towards a greater proportion of elderly individuals, traditional family structures must adapt to accommodate aging relatives. This transformation often leads to a reversal of caregiving roles, where younger generations find themselves providing support for their aging parents or grandparents. Such shifts can strain familial relationships and require adjustments in household dynamics. Communities are challenged to foster environments that promote social inclusion and active participation of older adults. Programs that encourage intergenerational engagements, such as community centers and volunteer initiatives, help diminish the isolation often associated with aging. The need for these initiatives is underscored by the observation that the aging population will require significant adjustments in how we structure our social services, healthcare systems, and community support networks *"As the population ages, there will be significant social and economic implications. The aging population will lead to a shift in the workforce, with older workers potentially staying in the workforce longer, and this could impact the job market and social security systems." (Linda P. Fried)*. Thus, understanding these interactions is pivotal for facilitating a harmonious coexistence across generations. Navigating the economic implications of an aging populace presents significant challenges and opportunities that affect societal structures. As people live longer, their needs and contributions to the workforce evolve, resulting in a demand for policies that support extended working lives. This phenomenon can lead to a reimagining of retirement age, as older adults remain active participants in the labor force, potentially alleviating some pressures on social security systems. Nevertheless, there is a growing concern regarding how this shift might impact younger workers, as competition for jobs may increase, creating economic friction. The workforce landscape may need to be restructured to balance the inclusion of various age groups effectively. Such socioeconomic dynamics underscore the hypothesis that as the population ages, there will be significant social and economic implications, ultimately emphasizing the need for adaptable economic policies that cater to the realities of an aging society. Societal attitudes towards aging will also play a crucial role in shaping the experiences of the elderly as life expectancy increases. Cultural perceptions about age and the value of older adults significantly influence their social roles and participation in community life. Societies that embrace aging as a phase of potential rather than decline tend to foster environments where older adults can thrive, contributing their knowledge and experience to a diverse array of sectors. Acceptance of this demographic shift is essential for promoting a holistic understanding of health and well-being in older age, which includes addressing issues such as ageism and promoting policies that enhance quality of life. The importance of addressing these cultural dimensions is clear; as the aging population continues to grow, developing a societal framework that values the contributions of elderly individuals will be critical in ensuring a cohesive and supportive environment for all ages. In essence, the social dynamics of an aging population compel us to rethink conventional norms surrounding work, family, and community, paving the way for a more inclusive future.

Changing Family Structures

As societal expectations shift in response to increasing life expectancies, it becomes essential to examine how family dynamics are evolving. The traditional nuclear family structure is being redefined as longer life spans encourage multigenerational living arrangements. In such configurations, wisdom from older generations can directly influence child-rearing practices, fostering stable environments conducive to healthy development. This interplay between age groups highlights the advantages of extensive familial networks that might provide emotional, psychological, and financial support when navigating the complexities of modern life. The impacts of such changes can contribute to a greater understanding of individual identities, encouraging adaptability among family members as they adjust to a world where extended ages become the norm. As noted, as people live longer, family structures are likely to change in significant ways, suggesting that these shifts will influence not just familial relationships but also societal expectations and norms. This transition warrants careful consideration of our preparedness for potential realities of living longer lives and their implications on family structures. Developments in technology and healthcare advancements also play a critical role in reshaping family dynamics. Emerging innovations, such as regenerative medicine and biotechnology, may enhance the quality of longevity by allowing individuals to maintain their health and vitality longer. Consequently, families might find themselves re-evaluating their roles and relationships as individuals increasingly defy the conventional limitations of aging. Elders, who once adopted more passive roles due to declining health, can now actively participate in family life, contributing to familial economies and cultural continuity. These shifts provide younger generations with valuable perspectives and experiences, which can aid in cultural transmission and social cohesion. Acknowledging these changes is crucial, as the re-envisioning of family roles could lead to both positive and negative repercussions for family life, requiring adaptive strategies to navigate the complexities introduced by longer life spans. Examining the broader societal implications reveals additional nuances surrounding changing family structures. As the concept of family diversifies, including single-parent households, child-free couples, and communal living arrangements, it becomes clear that the definition of family is evolving. This change will likely necessitate policy adjustments in areas such as healthcare, taxation, and social security to accommodate new family configurations that extend beyond traditional models. Understanding that each family structure carries unique challenges and strengths can inform public discourse and foster a more inclusive society. Acknowledging these diverse family types also emphasizes the need for community support systems that cater to various configurations, ultimately promoting reconciliation of responsibilities among family members. To appropriately address the implications of these shifts, it is vital to cultivate an understanding that the roles of grandparents and great-grandparents could evolve, ultimately enhancing societal adaptation strategies in response to longevity and changing family structures.

Intergenerational Relationships

The complexity of intergenerational relationships is accentuated as advancements in longevity extend life expectancies, prompting a reevaluation of familial and societal dynamics. As individuals live longer, the time spent across different generations is increasingly significant, creating opportunities for mutual support and shared experiences. This shift can foster a richer exchange of knowledge and values, bridging the generational divide. It also raises questions about the adaptability of societal structures to accommodate aging populations. Older adults often possess a wealth of experience and historical context that can greatly benefit younger generations, while the latter can provide technological prowess and fresh perspectives. The fusion of these attributes can lead to innovative solutions to pressing societal challenges, reinforcing the idea that healthy intergenerational relationships can positively influence community resilience. As noted, As people live longer, the relationships between generations become more complex and multifaceted, highlighting the necessity of understanding these evolving dynamics *"As people live longer, the relationships between generations become more complex and multifaceted. Understanding these dynamics is crucial for building supportive and inclusive societies." (Laura L. Carstensen)*. Nurturing intergenerational relationships plays a critical role in addressing the emotional and social needs of an aging population. These bonds can significantly alleviate feelings of isolation and loneliness that many older adults face. In contemporary society, where mobility and technology often limit personal interactions, fostering connections between generations becomes essential. Structured environments, such as community centers and educational workshops, can facilitate these interactions by bringing together younger and older individuals to engage in shared activities. Such platforms allow for the exchange of stories, skills, and perspectives, enhancing emotional wellbeing and enriching lives on both ends of the spectrum. These interactions can help debunk stereotypes about aging, promoting a more compassionate understanding of the challenges faced by older adults. The importance of lifestyle choices further emphasizes that nurturing intergenerational relationships can lead to shared learning experiences that promote healthful aging across all stages of life. Emerging research into the biological and psychological aspects of aging reinforces the significance of intergenerational relationships in promoting healthy development throughout life. Concepts such as the epigenetic clock and psychological resilience suggest that the quality of social interactions can lead to improved health outcomes and longevity. As older individuals maintain active engagement in their communities, they not only enhance their own wellbeing but also contribute positively to the health of younger generations. Engaging younger individuals in acts of service, mentorship, or even care for older adults creates an interdependent relationship that benefits all parties involved. These dynamics can generate a sense of purpose in older adults while instilling values of respect and care in younger generations. As societies prepare for longer life spans, encouraging intergenerational relationships can emerge as a potent strategy to enhance individual and collective quality of life. The synergy between aging populations and youth stands as a testament to the potential for building supportive relationships that foster both longevity and thriving societal structures; thus illustrating the importance of proactively cultivating these connections as we navigate the complexities of extended lifespans.

Community Support Systems

Acknowledging the profound implications of extended life expectancy necessitates a parallel examination of community support systems that can sustain individuals throughout their potentially lengthened lives. Strong community networks provide not only emotional support but also practical assistance that promotes overall well-being. As the demographic landscape evolves due to advancements in biotechnology and healthcare, communities will need to adapt their resources to cater to an increasingly aging population. This adaptation may manifest through established programs focusing on mental and physical wellness, which are critical as individuals face the complexities of aging. As articulated in the concept of social relationships as a significant factor for health outcomes, *"Social relationships, or the relative lack thereof, constitute a major risk factor for health—rivaling the effect of well-established health risk factors such as smoking, blood pressure, and physical activity." (Holt-Lunstad, J., Smith, T. B., & Layton, J. B.)*. The focus on community support systems is pivotal in ensuring that the advancements in longevity contribute positively to the quality of life in older age. The framework provided by community support systems extends well beyond mere social interactions; it includes access to healthcare services, recreational activities, and educational programs tailored to older adults. These services are essential for fostering engagement and maintaining an active lifestyle, countering the isolation that often accompanies aging.

Initiatives that promote lifelong learning not only stimulate cognitive function but also help maintain social connections, thus reinforcing a sense of belonging within the community. Programs that utilize technologies to monitor health and provide telemedicine services can effectively enhance these support systems, making healthcare more accessible. In this context, the exploration of emerging fields like regenerative medicine and genetic editing must align with community-driven initiatives that prioritize well-being alongside extended lifespans. Such integration underscores the necessity of adjusting societal structures to accommodate an aging population, ensuring that support systems evolve in tandem with health advancements. The role of community support systems is instrumental in addressing the ethical and economic challenges associated with increased longevity. As societies grapple with the implications of living significantly longer lives, the responsibility of intergenerational support intensifies. Communities can act as facilitators in bridging the gap between different age groups, fostering relationships that promote mutual assistance and understanding. As the labor market adjusts to accommodate older workers, community-based programs can help in retraining and integrating seniors into the workforce, thereby benefiting the economy. These initiatives help create a sustainable framework that not only nurtures the elderly but also empowers them as contributors to society. By uniting various elements within community support systems, societies can effectively prepare for the complexities associated with extended life expectancy, ultimately leading to more resilient, supportive environments for individuals across all age groups.

XII. CULTURAL PERSPECTIVES ON AGING

Cultural frameworks play a pivotal role in shaping attitudes towards aging and the elderly. In many societies, cultural narratives considerably influence how aging is perceived, often dictating respect, roles, and responsibilities associated with older individuals. In Eastern cultures, elder members are revered as repositories of wisdom and tradition, fostering a sense of familial and societal obligation toward their care. This contrasts sharply with Western paradigms, where aging is often associated with vulnerability and dependency, leading to a tendency to marginalize elderly individuals. Such cultural dichotomies indicate that societal respect for aging individuals not only affects personal interactions but can also impact policies regarding healthcare and social support systems. By understanding these cultural contrasts, we gain insights into how different societies might adapt to the long-term implications of an aging population, particularly as advancements in longevity science challenge traditional notions of age and elderhood. Aging is not merely a personal journey; it is profoundly influenced by social constructs that dictate how different cultures address the challenges and opportunities that come with an extended lifespan. Communities may differ significantly in their approaches to health, familial obligations, and institutional support for the elderly. The notion of filial piety in Asian cultures emphasizes the duty of children to care for their parents, creating a strong family-oriented model of aging. Conversely, in more individualistic cultures, retirement and elderly care may lean towards institutional settings, reflecting a societal shift in responsibility. This divergence becomes increasingly significant as longevity becomes a reality; societies with robust familial structures may navigate extended lifespans more gracefully than those that rely heavily on institutional frameworks. Through a comparative analysis of these sociocultural dimensions, we can address how collective societal norms shape individual experiences of aging, thereby influencing the adaptation to future longevity advancements. Examining cultural perceptions of aging is not only relevant for understanding societal attitudes but also crucial for considering the ethical implications of life-extension technologies. As developments in biotechnology and regenerative medicine present society with the potential to significantly prolong life, diverse cultural attitudes towards aging will determine the acceptance and integration of such technologies. Cultures that honor elder wisdom may prioritize technologies that enhance the quality of life and cognitive function in older age, while others might approach advancements with skepticism, fearing loss of autonomy or dignity. This interplay between cultural values and technological innovation necessitates dialogue around bioethics and societal roles in shaping policies related to aging. Image illustrates these long-term health challenges and mechanisms of aging, emphasizing the need for a culturally-informed approach to health interventions. Considering these cultural perspectives will be imperative for framing policies that not only address the medical aspects of longevity but also respect and acknowledge the diverse experiences and values associated with aging in a global context.

Variations in Attitudes Across Cultures

Cultural attitudes towards aging and longevity are profoundly shaped by historical, social, and economic factors, which can lead to varied perceptions of what it means to live a longer life. In many Western societies, the extension of life is often viewed through a lens of individualism, where advancements in healthcare are celebrated as personal achievements. This mindset tends to prioritize technology and innovation as the primary means to improve life expectancy, equating longevity with success and quality of life. Conversely, in numerous Eastern cultures, aging is often associated with wisdom and reverence for experience. Here, longer life is not solely a matter of medical advancement but also a cultural imperative that fosters intergenerational relationships and communal ties. As such, understanding these divergent perspectives is crucial, as they directly inform discussions surrounding the implications of living to 150, influencing social policies and healthcare resource allocation. Disparate cultural beliefs further manifest in how various societies perceive the quality of life associated with longevity. The increasing emphasis on mental health as a critical component of well-being is more pronounced in some cultures than others. While Western cultures might critique the aging process for its physical decline, prompting desires to inhibit times effects through medical intervention, other cultures may embrace aging as a stage of life that can be enriched through community support and holistic lifestyle practices. This contrasts sharply with the Western emphasis on anti-aging technologies, as explored through frameworks such as precision medicine and genetic editing, which are often underpinned by commercial interests. Understanding how these differing attitudes can influence health behaviors and policy responses is essential in preparing for the societal shifts that accompany longer lifespans, promoting engagement with cultural values and health beliefs to foster inclusive approaches to aging. The nexus between cultural perspectives and longevity underscores the necessity for a nuanced conversation about life extensions implications. Research into biological aging and interdisciplinary approaches, as seen in integrated studies spanning historical and molecular biology (as referenced in), can inform policies that are sensitive to the cultural contexts of healthcare practices. This aligned perspective is especially pertinent as societies grapple with conflicting views on the consequences of extending life. As discussions surrounding longevity continue to evolve, recognizing and respecting the variations in cultural attitudes will be vital in fostering acceptance of emerging technologies. Emphasizing a comprehensive understanding of these dynamics may enable societies to not only embrace the possibilities of living to 150 but to do so in a manner that resonates deeply with their cultural values and aspirations.

Country	Positive Attitude (%)	Neutral Attitude (%)	Negative Attitude (%)
Japan	82	12	6
United States	75	15	10
Germany	70	20	10
Brazil	65	25	10
India	80	15	5
China	78	18	4
Sweden	85	10	5
South Africa	72	20	8

Cultural Attitudes Toward Longevity

Rituals and Traditions Surrounding Aging

Cultural practices surrounding aging serve as a critical lens through which societies shape their understanding of life's later stages. Various regions have developed unique rituals that signify the transition into older age, influencing both personal identity and societal value. The Japanese tradition of Kanreki celebrates turning 60, symbolizing a new beginning and recognition of wisdom accumulated over a lifetime. Such practices highlight the importance of honoring elders and acknowledging the contributions they have made to their families and communities. Through these rituals, cultures provide frameworks that not only celebrate longevity but also reinforce the sense of purpose and belonging among older adults. This intertwining of aging with cultural identity provides insight into how societies can better appreciate and integrate aging individuals into the social fabric, potentially easing the transition into longer life spans as the concept of aging evolves. Exploring the multifaceted relationship between aging and societal rituals reveals significant implications for how we will navigate the future of longevity. As advancements in biotechnology and regenerative medicine present the possibility of extending human life beyond previous limits, the existing traditions surrounding aging will inevitably evolve. Cultures that actively engage in honoring the elderly, such as through communal storytelling or mentorship programs, may find themselves better positioned to adapt to these changes. Traditions that incorporate elders perspectives into community decision-making processes can enhance intergenerational dialogue, ensuring that the insights gained from longer life experiences are not lost. As seen in diagrams showcasing systems biology and aging mechanisms, understanding these connections can empower societies to cultivate rites of passage that keep pace with scientific progress while fostering respect and integration of older adults into community life. The ethical challenges associated with longevity also intersect with rituals and traditions. A society that increasingly prioritizes extending life must simultaneously confront the question of how to maintain dignity, respect, and quality of life for aging individuals. Many cultures have established end-of-life rituals that encourage reflection and honor the life lived, seen in practices that emphasize gratitude and closure. As life expectancy potentially extends to 150 years, there will be a critical need to adapt these traditions to reflect new realities, allowing for celebrations of life while also addressing the complexities of prolonged aging. This evolving paradigm can serve as a soil for new rituals that simultaneously honor the past and embrace the future, leading to a more profound understanding of aging, as depicted in scientific frameworks analyzing health and interventional strategies. Integrating ethical considerations with emerging rituals can foster a culture that respects aging while embracing new lifestyles and technologies.

Global Perspectives on Longevity

The conversation surrounding longevity is not merely scientific; it is inherently social, intertwining with cultural norms and societal values globally. Different countries exhibit varying perceptions of aging, which significantly impacts their policy approaches and health initiatives. In many Western societies, aging is often viewed through a deficit lens, focusing on the challenges of care and health decline. Conversely, certain Eastern cultures may celebrate the wisdom and experience associated with older age, integrating elderly members into family units and communities more holistically. This divergence becomes particularly evident when considering healthcare policies. As some argue that advances in medicine and technology could significantly enhance life expectancy, Measurable disparities arise in how societies address older adults needs. This illustrates the complex interplay between culture and the practical implications of longevity initiatives. Understanding global perspectives on aging is imperative for crafting effective policies that honor both individual dignity and communal interdependence. As longevity becomes a more tangible possibility, significant ethical concerns emerge regarding resource allocation and societal impacts. Challenges such as healthcare access, economic sustainability, and quality of life for older adults must be addressed vigorously. The notion of living longer holds promise but also raises questions about the implications of extended life on resources and social structures. The sustainability of pension systems and healthcare resources could be compromised by a burgeoning population of older adults. As one scholar remarked, The global perspective on longevity is multifaceted, involving not just the biological and medical aspects but also the social, economic, and cultural implications of increased lifespan. These implications necessitate a re-evaluation of existing systems and cultural interpretations of aging. In recognizing the multifaceted dimensions of longevity, societies can work towards equitable solutions that promote health, well-being, and dignity throughout the lifespan. A significant aspect of longevity discussions involves evolving scientific and technological innovations that could alter the trajectory of human aging. Fields such as biotechnology and regenerative medicine hold transformative potential, offering unprecedented opportunities to enhance health and extend life. These innovations require careful scrutiny regarding ethical considerations and potential societal ramifications. The development of aging clocks and health biomarkers can provide insights into individual aging processes, facilitating personalized approaches to health management. Embracing such advancements necessitates addressing disparities in access to these technologies, ensuring that benefits are distributed equitably across populations. The evolving landscape of healthcare also demands that societies reconsider traditional familial structures and roles. New models of care will be essential in a world where living beyond 100 may be commonplace. Thus, exploring these scientific advancements alongside cultural and social dynamics is critical for preparing for a future characterized by significant increases in longevity.

Country	Life Expectancy (Years)	Healthy Life Expectancy (Years)
Japan	84.6	74.5
Switzerland	83.5	73.5
Australia	83.4	73.9
Singapore	84.2	74.9
Spain	83.2	73.3
Italy	83.3	74.1
Canada	82.4	72.5
France	82.9	72.4
United States	78.9	68
Germany	81.3	71

Global Longevity Statistics by Country (2023)

XIII. POLICY CONSIDERATIONS FOR LONGEVITY

In considering longevity, policymakers must grapple with the shifting landscape of public health and the potential strain on existing healthcare systems. As research progresses in fields like regenerative medicine and biotechnology, it becomes crucial to evaluate how such advancements will be integrated into current health infrastructures. A major concern lies in the accessibility and affordability of these innovations. If the technologies designed to extend life are only available to a privileged few, this could exacerbate existing socioeconomic disparities. Additionally, how interpersonal relationships and community support structures adapt to increased longevity needs careful examination. Community healthcare initiatives will need to evolve not just to treat age-related diseases but also to promote wellness across longer life spans. This consideration underscores the necessity for policies that prioritize equitable access to healthcare advancements, facilitating broader benefits rather than deepening societal divides. The insights in about applications of Deep Generative Reinforcement Learning highlight how innovative approaches can enhance biomedical research, supporting the case for policy adaptation. Another aspect of longevity policy involves the restructuring of societal frameworks to accommodate an aging population. Current systems are largely predicated on conventional life expectancies, and a shift towards longer lives necessitates rethinking retirement age, workforce participation, and social services. Extending working years may require flexibility in employment practices, where older adults are allowed to contribute based on their capacities. Alongside this, educational systems may need to offer lifelong learning opportunities to ensure that individuals remain engaged and productive throughout extended lifespans. As illustrated in, dietary habits and nutrition play a key role in health across the lifespan and are essential to longevity. Policymaking must therefore incorporate aspects of public health education that promote healthy lifestyles and nutrition, aiming to improve quality of life as life expectancy increases. The transition to a society that embraces the longevity revolution will involve significant adjustments across multiple sectors, underscoring the importance of visionary policies that challenge conventional frameworks. Ethical considerations surrounding longevity cannot be overlooked, as advancements in genetic editing and biotechnology prompt essential moral inquiries. Determining who has the right to access life-extending technologies raises significant ethical dilemmas; equitable distribution must be a paramount goal in policy development. Additionally, there are questions regarding the impact of prolonged life on planetary sustainability and resource allocation. As indicated in, the multi-omic approaches play a crucial role in understanding aging but also emphasize the need for responsible research and application. Balancing the benefits of extended life with the potential for overpopulation and environmental degradation leads to a complex landscape for policymakers. It is imperative that discussions around longevity policies are inclusive, engaging experts from ethics, ecology, and economics to ensure the creation of sustainable and equitable systems. Integrating these considerations will be crucial for successfully navigating the societal implications of living to 150 years and beyond.

Year	Country	Life Expectancy	Public Spending On Health	Pension Expenditure
2020	United States	78.54	10,965	8.5
2021	United States	78.99	11,525	8.7
2022	United States	79.11	12,100	9
2023	United States	79.5	12,750	9.2

Policy Considerations for Longevity Statistics

Government Regulations on Biotechnology

The regulatory landscape surrounding biotechnology is a complex integration of laws and guidelines designed to ensure public safety, foster innovation, and address ethical dilemmas. As biotechnological advancements accelerate, so too does the necessity for robust government oversight. Agencies like the Food and Drug Administration (FDA) in the United States play a pivotal role in evaluating the safety and efficacy of biotechnological products. Regulatory frameworks must adapt continuously to keep pace with innovations such as CRISPR gene editing, synthetic biology, and regenerative medicine. Without meticulous regulations, the potential for misuse or unintended consequences increases, raising existential questions about bioethics and human dignity. The challenge, therefore, lies in striking a balance between encouraging scientific progress and safeguarding public health and environmental sustainability. This dynamic interplay will significantly influence the trajectory of biotechnology and its role in extending human longevity. serves as a reliable visual guide in this context, elucidating various biological mechanisms of aging with relevance to biotechnological applications and regulatory considerations. Numerous challenges arise when implementing government regulations on biotechnology, particularly concerning ethical implications and public perception. The potential for genetic modifications, whether in agricultural systems or human therapeutics, elicits diverse attitudes among stakeholders, ranging from apprehension to enthusiastic acceptance. This diversity often complicates the regulatory process, as policymakers endeavor to balance scientific advancement with ethical boundaries. The influence of lobby groups, advocacy organizations, and public sentiment cannot be overlooked; each plays a vital role in shaping perceptions of biotechnological innovations. As biotechnological advancements increasingly permeate societal structures, regulations must remain transparent and adaptable, addressing ethical concerns such as informed consent, environmental impact, and equity in access. Image highlights this relationship by illustrating how various applications of biotechnology intersect with governmental oversight, reflecting the increasing relevance of regulations as innovations in aging sciences progress. Preparing for a future where biotechnology significantly contributes to human longevity necessitates a nuanced understanding of regulatory frameworks across global contexts. Different countries exhibit varying degrees of regulatory stringency, informed by cultural attitudes toward biotechnology and risk. European Union regulations on genetically modified organisms (GMOs) are famously stricter than those in the United States, reflecting broader societal consent toward safety and environmental sustainability. These differences pose challenges for international collaboration and may hinder innovations that could streamline healthcare and enhance quality of life. Additionally, emerging technologies in synthetic biology and genetic editing require a global dialogue, promoting harmonized regulations that protect public health while fostering innovation. Without such cooperative frameworks, geographic disparities in access to advanced biotechnological solutions for longevity may lead to heightened inequalities. The implications of these regulations are vital for shaping future societal dynamics, making an understanding of international policy landscapes essential for anyone engaged in biotechnology. The comprehensive examination provided by offers crucial insights into the multi-omic approach to aging, underlining the intersection of legislative measures and scientific inquiry in this rapidly evolving field.

Public Health Initiatives

In examining the landscape of health outcomes, the role of public health initiatives becomes paramount, shaping our understanding of longevity and quality of life. These initiatives often serve as a bridge connecting the advances in medical technology with the broader socio-economic factors that influence health. Successful public health campaigns have been crucial in combating chronic diseases linked to aging, such as diabetes and heart disease. By addressing lifestyle factors like diet and exercise through community outreach and education, these programs foster a more health-conscious society that can mitigate some of the detrimental effects of extended lifespans. As health determinants evolve, understanding their multifaceted nature is essential; this complexity can be visualized through frameworks that emphasize interconnected biological and sociocultural factors. The development of such frameworks highlights the necessity for public health to adapt continually, ensuring that longevity is accompanied by a high quality of life for all. New approaches to health monitoring and assessment, such as those illustrated by age-related biological markers, are becoming increasingly integral to public health strategies aimed at extending lifespans. One significant focus is on understanding aging at a cellular and molecular level, utilizing insights from emerging fields like biotechnology. Public health initiatives can leverage these discoveries to promote preventive health measures and personalized medicine. As noted in recent studies, the urgency of reducing greenhouse gas emissions became increasingly evident, a reflection of how interconnected environmental factors and health outcomes are, thus emphasizing the necessity of environmentally focused public health policies. By integrating knowledge from molecular biology into preventive health programs, we can foster environments that not only support health but actively promote longevity. This synthesis of science and policy showcases the potential of public health initiatives to significantly influence life expectancy and overall well-being. In thinking about the future of longevity, public health initiatives must also consider the ethical implications of extended lifespans on societal structures. The longevity revolution brings forward questions about resource distribution, healthcare access, and cultural perceptions of aging. Initiatives that focus on equitable health access are crucial to ensure that prolonged life is not confined to specific demographics but is universally beneficial. Integrating public health frameworks with community engagement strategies can address disparities by tailoring interventions to meet the cultural and socio-economic dynamics of diverse populations. Consequently, analyzing how different cultures approach aging reveals both challenges and opportunities. Cultivating a comprehensive understanding of aging through a public health lens allows for the creation of inclusive policies that embrace the complexities of an aging population. This approach not only optimizes health outcomes but also nurtures intergenerational dynamics within society, ultimately preparing us for the reality of living significantly longer lives.

Initiative	Year	Impact on Longevity	Source
Vaccination Programs	2023	Increase by 3-5 years	World Health Organization (WHO)
Smoking Cessation Programs	2023	Increase by 7-10 years	Centers for Disease Control and Prevention (CDC)
Obesity Prevention Campaigns	2023	Increase by 2-4 years	National Institute of Health (NIH)
Mental Health Awareness	2023	Increase by 2-3 years	American Psychological Association (APA)
Chronic Disease Management Programs	2023	Increase by 5-7 years	American Heart Association (AHA)

Public Health Initiatives Impact on Longevity

Funding for Aging Research

The complexities of aging research demand adequate funding to explore and implement innovative solutions that can enhance longevity and quality of life. Investment in this field is crucial, particularly as the global population ages and the associated health challenges grow. Despite the significance of such research, funding sources often remain inconsistent, relying heavily on governmental support and private sponsorships. Programs like the National Institute on Aging (NIA) focus on developing age-related research initiatives, yet they face financial limitations that can hinder groundbreaking studies. Without a robust funding framework, the potential advancements in regenerative medicine and biotechnology may remain unrealized, ultimately affecting the holistic understanding of aging processes. As highlighted in, a conceptual framework outlining biological mechanisms of aging emphasizes that sustained investment can promote significant discoveries. Stakeholders must prioritize the allocation of resources to aging research to ensure that society can effectively address the health issues linked to increased longevity. Transitioning from basic research to practical applications necessitates that funding mechanisms adapt to the evolving landscape of aging science. Emphasizing systems biology, which integrates multi-omic approaches to understand aging, illustrates how complex biological interactions can inform therapeutic strategies. The current funding paradigms, however, often prioritize short-term outputs over long-term impact, potentially stymying transformative advancements in health outcomes. As depicted in, the integration of various omics can yield valuable insights that propel aging research forward. A shift in funding strategies could encourage interdisciplinary collaboration, uniting experts from fields such as genetics, bioinformatics, and public health to cultivate a more comprehensive understanding of aging. By aligning financial support with the multifaceted nature of aging, researchers can pioneer holistic interventions that promise to improve the quality of life for an increasingly aging population. Public perception and cultural attitudes towards aging significantly influence funding opportunities. Societal attitudes in cultures that embrace longevity, as opposed to those that view aging as a decline, can affect the prioritization of aging research funding. Engaging the public through awareness campaigns can stimulate interest in approaching aging not merely as a biological process but as a holistic experience that warrants exploration and innovation. Addressing public misconceptions about aging is pivotal to fostering a supportive environment for funding agencies. As illustrated in, diverse influences of dietary practices on healthy aging elucidate the importance of understanding lifestyle factors in longevity research. Consequently, funding initiatives that prioritize community engagement and cultural relevance can amplify resources directed toward comprehensive aging studies, ensuring that advancements align with the societal needs and aspirational challenges of longevity.

XIV. ENVIRONMENTAL SUSTAINABILITY AND LONGEVITY

Environmental sustainability plays a pivotal role in the pursuit of longevity, especially as the global population anticipates life spans extending toward 150 years. Urbanization, industrialization, and unsustainable resource extraction threaten ecosystems, leading to implications for human health and longevity. Environmental degradation has been linked to numerous health crises, such as respiratory diseases, cardiovascular issues, and infectious diseases, all of which severely affect the quality and length of life. A focus on sustainable practices, such as renewable energy use, eco-friendly agriculture, and pollution reduction, can mitigate these risks. By fostering interconnected practices that support both human health and the environment, communities can build resilience against diseases that may become more prevalent in an aging population. Incorporating this holistic perspective is essential, as it recognizes that the environment and individual health are mutually influential and underscores the importance of proactive measures to sustain health over lengthy life spans. Emerging technologies are increasingly viewed as integral to environmental sustainability, driving innovative solutions aimed at improving quality of life as we age. Advances in biotechnology, such as genetically engineered crops that require fewer resources, aim to enhance food security while reducing environmental strain. Similarly, regenerative medicine leverages natural processes to repair or replace damaged tissues or organs, potentially extending healthy life years while minimizing ecological footprints. By enhancing our biological systems—both in health and in agriculture—these technologies also contribute to the sustainability of food systems and environmental resilience, ensuring that as lifespans lengthen, we mitigate the adverse effects of overpopulation and resource depletion. Integrating sustainable practices within these scientific advancements aligns longevity goals with environmental stewardship, creating a pathway for a future where health and ecological balance coexist harmoniously. As outlined in, the interplay of nutritional approaches and aging provides a foundational understanding of how healthier eating, influenced by sustainable practices, can contribute to overall well-being and longevity. The cultural dimensions of environmental sustainability significantly influence societal attitudes towards longevity. Different cultures prioritize sustainability in varying degrees, with some recognizing intrinsic links between environmental health and community well-being. Cultures that incorporate traditional ecological knowledge often champion sustainable practices as a means to preserve both the environment and the quality of life for future generations. Such cultural norms dictate not only how resources are utilized but also how aging populations are viewed and supported within the community framework. Policies that promote sustainability can also foster intergenerational solidarity, as older and younger community members work together to create livable environments. This cultural synergy enhances social fabric and contributes to the holistic health of the population, reinforcing the need for policies that embrace both sustainability and longevity as interdependent goals. As indicated in, understanding the determinants of health in relation to this framework provides clarity on the objectives needed to align health policies with sustainable community development.

Year	Average Life Expectancy (Years)	CO2 Emissions Per Capita (Tons)	Countries with Sustainable Practices (%)
2020	78.8	16.1	30
2021	79.1	15.5	32
2022	79.6	14.7	34
2023	79.9	14.2	36

Environmental Sustainability and Longevity Statistics

Resource Management for an Aging Population

Meeting the challenges posed by an aging population requires a multifaceted approach to resource management that addresses both immediate and long-term needs. This demographic shift emphasizes the necessity for a coordinated healthcare system that integrates preventative care, ongoing management of chronic conditions, and supportive services tailored to the elderly. Innovations in deep generative reinforcement learning, as highlighted in, showcase how data-driven approaches can enhance capabilities like biological age prediction and precision medicine, thus allowing healthcare providers to allocate resources more efficiently. By understanding individual health trajectories, proactive measures can be implemented, improving quality of life while potentially reducing healthcare expenditures. This focus on preventive strategies is paramount as it shifts the healthcare paradigm from reactive to proactive care, ensuring that resources are used not merely to manage diseases, but to maintain the overall well-being of older adults. Economic sustainability alongside healthcare adaptation is critical for managing an aging population effectively. As life expectancy increases, societies must adapt their economic frameworks to support longer lifespans through policies aimed at retirement, pensions, and labor force participation. Emphasizing the importance of integrative longevity strategies, illustrates how multi-omic approaches in understanding aging can inform economic decisions. By recognizing the intricate biological and social factors that contribute to health in advanced age, policymakers can design interventions that promote inclusion and productivity among older adults. This approach can mitigate potential economic burdens while fostering a more robust labor market. Enabling older individuals to contribute to society and the economy not only addresses challenges associated with an increasing dependency ratio but also underscores the value of their experiences and skills. Tackling the resource management dilemmas inherent in an aging demographic calls for innovative strategies that embrace interdisciplinary collaboration. The integration of various fields, such as biotechnology, social sciences, and gerontology, is essential for developing effective solutions to complex challenges. The diagram presented in underscores the importance of addressing systemic, cellular, and molecular changes in aging as part of a cohesive resource management plan. Understanding these layers contributes to holistic health strategies that enhance accessibility to essential services while promoting intergenerational bonds. By encouraging collaborative frameworks that involve community participation, governments, and healthcare providers, societies can foster environments that support aging populations effectively. This holistic perspective is vital as it prepares communities to thrive amidst the demographic trends, ensuring that all individuals have the resources they need to lead fulfilling lives as they age.

Impact of Longevity on Climate Change

As society progresses toward extended life expectancies, there is an imperative to consider the ecological implications of a growing population, particularly in relation to sustainability. Prolonged human longevity may lead to increased resource consumption, intensified waste generation, and heightened pressure on our planet's ecosystems. The potential influx of older individuals into an already strained socioeconomic framework poses questions about environmental sustainability. As highlighted in, dietary approaches that focus on healthy aging not only enhance individual well-being but also minimize ecological footprints. Transitioning to sustainable eating patterns can mitigate some adverse environmental impacts associated with increased longevity, promoting an interconnected approach that values both health and ecological stewardship. Planning for longer lifespans necessitates a dual focus on human health and the preservation of natural resources, encouraging innovative solutions that reconcile the two spheres for future sustainable living. An aging population demands re-evaluation of urban planning and resource allocation, especially as older citizens typically require more healthcare services. This demographic shift can exacerbate existing environmental challenges, such as urban sprawl and carbon emissions from transportation associated with healthcare access. The interrelation between age-related healthcare needs and environmental sustainability is complex, as the rise in chronic illnesses often necessitates greater healthcare infrastructure, which in turn contributes to greenhouse gas emissions. Tools and models illustrated in emphasize how ecological practices can be integrated into healthcare systems, promoting sustainability while catering to the needs of an aging populace. Fostering age-friendly environments, paired with innovative age-related technologies, can ease the strain on resources, aligning healthcare practices with sustainable development goals. This holistic approach will not only support healthy aging but also curtail the environmental footprint associated with healthcare service delivery. The influence of longevity on climate change extends to social dynamics and intergenerational relationships, as longer life expectancy leads to the possibility of multiple generations coexisting over extended periods. This demographic shift could challenge traditional family structures and societal roles, necessitating adaptations that enable resource-sharing and climate action across age groups. Older adults often possess valuable knowledge and experience that can inform sustainable practices, as portrayed in the frameworks presented in. Engaging younger generations in dialogues with their elders can foster a collective sense of responsibility for the planet. Additionally, reshaping educational initiatives to address climate change will be vital, ensuring that all age groups understand the implications of their lifestyles on planetary health. By embracing an inclusive perspective on longevity that incorporates environmental considerations, society can work concurrently towards longevity and ecological preservation.

Year	Global Population	Average Life Expectancy	CO_2 Emissions Per Capita	Elderly Population (%)
2020	7.8 Billion	72.6 Years	4.8 Metric Tons	9.4
2025	8.1 Billion	73.7 Years	4.9 Metric Tons	10.3
2030	8.5 Billion	74.6 Years	5.1 Metric Tons	11.2
2035	8.8 Billion	75.4 Years	5.3 Metric Tons	12.1
2040	9.2 Billion	76.2 Years	5.5 Metric Tons	13.0

Impact of Longevity on Climate Change Indicators

Sustainable Practices for Long Life

In an era marked by rapid technological advancement, understanding the role of sustainability in promoting longevity is paramount. Sustainable practices not only ensure a healthier planet but also foster environments conducive to long life. Adopting a plant-based diet has been linked to reduced risks of chronic diseases, such as heart disease and diabetes, which are prevalent in aging populations. A thriving ecosystem supports food diversity, essential for nutrition and health, by maintaining soil fertility and preserving biodiversity. An image illustrating the relationships among various dietary approaches, such as the Mediterranean diet and caloric restriction, can underscore their impacts on healthy aging. By visually representing how these diets influence factors such as weight loss and inflammation, encapsulates the profound interrelationship between sustainable eating habits and enhanced longevity. Thus, pursuing sustainable dietary practices can pave the way for longer, healthier lives, reinforcing the notion that our choices significantly influence our health trajectories. In addition to dietary adjustments, the integration of technology in fostering sustainable practices plays a critical role in enhancing longevity. Advances in renewable energy sources and green living spaces can create environments that promote physical activity and mental well-being, essential components of a long life. Community designs that prioritize walkability and access to green spaces encourage outdoor activities, reducing sedentary lifestyles. Integrating smart technologies, such as monitors for air quality or tools that promote sustainable agricultural practices, can enhance community health. The relevance of these techniques is exemplified in, where the interconnectedness of different health determinants is visualized. The diagram emphasizes how various levels of the health domain—ranging from individual behavior to community health—interconnect in addressing the broad issues of aging and sustainability. By implementing tech-driven solutions within communities, we bolster public health and contribute to the overall longevity of populations. Addressing the environmental implications of prolonged life expectancy also necessitates sustainable public policy frameworks. Governments must invest in infrastructure that supports long-term health by focusing on sustainable resource management, waste reduction, and pollution control. Policies that promote urban farming, renewable energy, and green transportation options not only enhance public health but also reduce the ecological footprint of aging populations. Public awareness campaigns that educate citizens about sustainable practices can transform community attitudes towards health and longevity. The visual representation in illustrates the interplay between individual and societal health determinants, demonstrating the importance of comprehensive policies that integrate these dimensions. By fostering a culture that values sustainability, societies can ensure that as life expectancy increases, quality of life and environmental health improve in tandem, creating a viable future for generations to come.

XV. QUALITY OF LIFE IN OLD AGE

The pursuit of prolonged life raises critical considerations about the quality of life for the elderly. Advancements in healthcare and technology promise not only increased longevity but also the enhancement of well-being in old age. This perspective shifts the focus from mere survival to thriving in later years, emphasizing factors such as mental health, social connections, and access to healthcare. Innovations in fields like biotechnology and digital health tools are paving the way for individuals to manage chronic conditions more effectively and maintain a healthy lifestyle. Platforms that integrate health monitoring with mental health support can empower older adults to make informed decisions and lead fulfilling lives, directly addressing their quality of life. The intersection of these technologies and ongoing medical research catalyzes an environment where the elderly are encouraged to participate actively in their health management, thereby enhancing their overall experience in the later stages of life. A comprehensive understanding of quality of life in old age necessitates acknowledging the vital role of social engagement. As individuals age, maintaining social ties can significantly influence emotional well-being and cognitive health. Research has shown that loneliness and social isolation are prevalent among older adults, leading to detrimental health outcomes. Community support systems, including local programs and initiatives that foster camaraderie among seniors, can mitigate these effects and promote an active lifestyle. The potential for collaborative activities, such as group exercise or shared learning experiences, showcases the importance of community in ensuring that elderly individuals do not merely survive but thrive. Additionally, intergenerational relationships can be crucial, as they not only provide emotional support but also facilitate knowledge exchange, contributing to a richer quality of life. By prioritizing social engagement through targeted initiatives, society can better prepare for the reality of living longer lives. Advancing the quality of life in old age also involves grappling with ethical dilemmas and societal responsibilities. As we contemplate the implications of living potentially beyond 150 years, it becomes imperative to consider how resources will be allocated to support an aging population. This encompasses healthcare access, financial stability, and the provision of age-friendly environments. Policymakers and communities must work collaboratively to create sustainable systems that encompass both technological innovation and social facets to care for the elderly. The balance between enhancing individual health through technology and ensuring that societal structures support older adults is critical. In this context, the role of education becomes essential, as awareness and preparedness for aging must permeate all levels of society. By addressing these ethical considerations and societal challenges, we can aspire not only to extend life but to enhance the experience of living through quality engagement and shared resources.

Year	Country	Life Expectancy	Quality of Life Index	Population Aged 65 and Over
2020	United States	78.93	69.8	16.5
2020	Japan	84.64	83.6	28.7
2020	Germany	81.21	70.4	21.9
2020	Italy	83.21	76.5	23
2020	Sweden	82.52	77.9	20.3
2020	Canada	82.05	76	18.5
2020	Australia	82.9	79.4	16
2020	France	82.52	77.3	20.8
2020	United Kingdom	81.2	77	18.5
2020	Singapore	84.07	82.4	15.2

Quality of Life in Old Age

Defining Quality of Life

Quality of life encompasses a multifaceted array of dimensions that extend beyond mere survival or physical health. It involves not only the absence of disease but also the presence of holistic well-being that integrates physical, emotional, psychological, and social health. In assessing quality of life, one must consider factors such as mental health stability, life satisfaction, access to healthcare, social connections, and the ability to engage in enjoyable activities. As we contemplate extending human lifespans significantly, focusing solely on longevity without regard to these aspects of quality creates a paradox. The possibilities of living longer can become hollow if individuals endure chronic pain, isolation, or a lack of purpose. This interconnectedness between longevity and quality of life underscores the need for comprehensive strategies that encompass not just the extension of life but also enhancements in the quality of the life lived during those years. Increasingly, researchers are turning to technological advancements to facilitate improved quality of life for individuals as they age. Innovations in biotechnology and regenerative medicine are promising avenues that may help alleviate age-related ailments and enhance overall well-being. As highlighted in, understanding biological aging processes, such as genomic instability and altered intercellular communications, provides valuable insights into potential interventions that can significantly modify the aging trajectory. Tools such as deep generative reinforcement learning could play a role in personalized medicine, enabling targeted treatments that address the unique needs of diverse individual profiles. Such advancements create an opportunity not only to extend life but to enrich it, providing individuals with the capability to maintain independence, remain socially active, and engage in fulfilling activities that contribute to their sense of purpose and belonging. The social and cultural implications of a prolonged lifespan raise difficult questions about the definition of quality of life. Not all individuals or societies perceive aging or longevity in the same light. As seen in, the determinants of health are deeply rooted in social structures, and quality of life can vary considerably across different populations. Cultural attitudes towards aging, support systems within families, and community engagement all shape how individuals experience their later years. The pursuit of a longer life must therefore be accompanied by an inclusive dialogue about societal values and resources. Establishing frameworks that prioritize both physical health and emotional well-being fosters an environment where individuals can thrive, regardless of age. This holistic view not only enriches discussions around longevity but also aligns with the ethical imperative to ensure that extended years are meaningful and valuable for individuals and society alike.

Health span vs. Lifespan

The distinction between health span and lifespan represents a crucial consideration in discussions about longevity and the quality of life in an increasingly aged population. While lifespan refers to the total number of years a person lives, health span is defined as the duration of life spent in good health, free from chronic diseases and functional decline. This differentiation is essential, given the scientific advancements that promise to extend human life. Proponents of longevity research advocate for an increase in health span to ensure that individuals not only live longer but also maintain physical and mental vitality well into their later years. By prioritizing health span, we can shift the focus of public health policy from merely extending life to enhancing the quality of those additional years, fostering a society where older individuals contribute meaningfully without the burden of debilitating health issues. As we explore the implications of living up to 150 years, ensuring health span remains a focal point will be paramount. In examining the current landscape of health and aging, insights from groundbreaking research illuminate the multifaceted nature of health span. Integrative approaches such as those highlighted in the schematic representations in and underscore the interplay between genetic, environmental, and lifestyle factors in determining both lifespan and health span. The focus on systems biology reveals that aging is not merely a biological endpoint but an intricate web of interactions influenced by various determinants. By harnessing knowledge from fields such as biomedicine and gerontology, researchers are discovering ways to enhance health at the molecular and cellular levels, as illustrated in the studies of dietary interventions and their positive effects on health outcomes. The images collectively emphasize that while extending lifespan may seem like an alluring goal, the true challenge lies in ensuring that individuals can thrive healthily as they age, therefore making health span a more pressing issue in longevity discussions. Addressing the societal implications of extending longevity is equally important to understanding the balance between lifespan and health span. As portrayed in and, there are profound implications for healthcare systems, economic structures, and social relationships when considering how we define quality of life in older age. With an increasing number of individuals living longer, there will be heightened demand for medical services, supportive care, and community resources tailored to the needs of these populations. The prospect of prolonged life raises critical questions regarding sustainable healthcare practices and social equity. It invites a re-evaluation of current societal norms surrounding work, retirement, and caregiving, calling for innovative solutions that account for the unique experiences of an aging population. Exploring these dynamics will be essential in developing strategies that promote a balanced approach to longevity—one that prioritizes a meaningful, healthy existence rather than solely an extended chronological lifespan.

Age Group	Lifespan Average	Health span Average
0-20	78.5	78.5
21-40	78.5	76
41-60	78.5	70
61-80	78.5	65
81+	78.5	60

Health span vs. Lifespan Data

Enhancing Life Satisfaction

Achieving a sense of fulfillment is essential for enhancing life satisfaction, especially in the context of extended lifespans. As individuals live longer, the pursuit of meaningful experiences becomes a critical focus. Engaging in activities that promote personal growth, such as continued education or skill development, contributes significantly to an individual's sense of purpose. Studies have shown that lifelong learning not only stimulates cognitive function but also fosters social connections, which are key components of emotional well-being. Involvement in community service and volunteer efforts not only aids in personal development but enhances connectivity with others. These engagements instill a feeling of contribution and broader life meaning, crucial for navigating the psychological complexities associated with living extended years. As we explore the implications of longevity, understanding the vital role of personal fulfillment markers like education and community involvement can help frame support systems that foster life satisfaction in older adults. As enhancements in healthcare and technology continue to transform our lifestyles, examining how these advancements affect interpersonal relationships is necessary for understanding overall life satisfaction. Strengthening connections with family and friends becomes an increasingly critical aspect as people navigate long-lasting years. Research highlights that strong social networks contribute positively to both mental and emotional health, significantly mitigating feelings of isolation or loneliness that can arise in later life. The capacity to foster these connections is bolstered by advancements in communication technologies, which allow for greater interaction, even across physical distances. Video chatting platforms facilitate family gatherings and friendships that might otherwise diminish due to geographical separation. These technological innovations serve as an essential support system for individuals, ensuring that their social bonds remain intact, thereby enhancing their overall quality of life as they age. Integrating such communicative strategies not only enriches life satisfaction but also redefines how we engage with loved ones in an increasingly extended lifespan. Considering the implications of cultural attitudes towards aging and life satisfaction reveals significant variations across societies. Cultures that actively celebrate the elderly tend to foster environments where senior individuals feel valued and connected, thereby enhancing their overall life satisfaction. In many Asian cultures, the respect and reverence afforded to older generations create a profound sense of belonging and purpose. In contrast, cultures that marginalize the elderly can engender feelings of alienation and dissatisfaction, potentially leading to adverse mental health outcomes. Integrating insights from such cultural perspectives can inform policies and practices aimed at improving life satisfaction among aging populations. Understanding these cultural nuances can aid in devising interdisciplinary approaches that blend healthcare, community resources, and psychological support, ultimately promoting well-being during extended lifetimes. Embracing within the discourse of longevity the importance of respecting and valuing age can significantly reshape societal attitudes and practices, fostering a supportive environment for enhanced life satisfaction in the years ahead.

XVI. THE ROLE OF TECHNOLOGY IN ELDER CARE

Technological innovations are reshaping the landscape of elder care, making it possible to enhance the quality of life for aging individuals significantly. From telehealth services to wearable health monitors, these advancements provide invaluable support for managing chronic conditions and ensuring regular health assessments. Remote monitoring devices, for example, allow caregivers to track vital signs in real-time, facilitating timely interventions when health declines are detected. Such proactive measures are critical, as they enable a more personalized approach to care, wherein treatment plans can be adjusted based on immediate data rather than relying solely on scheduled appointments. This shift towards data-driven elder care exemplifies the broader trend of integrating technology to promote not just longevity, but also the overall well-being of elderly populations. The cultural implications of technology in elder care cannot be overlooked. As artificial intelligence-driven platforms emerge, they create opportunities for increased social engagement, combatting the isolation often faced by seniors. Virtual reality experiences allow elderly individuals to engage in immersive activities, from exploring distant locales to participating in group social activities with peers. Such innovations reflect the growing understanding that mental and emotional health is just as important as physical health in promoting quality of life. As one expert noted, with the help of artificial intelligence, we analyze the multivariate mass spectrometry data and multivariate vitalomics data to find the correlation between these complex data. This highlights the potential for technology not only to address the physical needs of the elderly but also to enhance their mental and emotional health through innovative engagement strategies. The integration of technology in elder care also raises ethical considerations that warrant careful examination. As families increasingly rely on tech solutions, the risk of reduced personal interaction arises, potentially eroding traditional caregiving roles. Issues related to data privacy and security are paramount, as sensitive health information becomes digitized and shared across platforms. As we navigate these challenges, it is essential to strike a balance between harnessing technological advancements and preserving the personal connections that are crucial for emotional support. The establishment of dedicated research initiatives, such as the National Key Laboratory of Chinese Medicine Syndrome, aims to explore these dynamics more comprehensively. By doing so, we can leverage technology in elder care while fostering an environment where human connections remain at the forefront, ultimately benefiting the aging population as they approach living longer, healthier lives.

Telehealth and Remote Monitoring

Recent advancements in technology have forged a path toward more accessible healthcare solutions, with telehealth and remote monitoring emerging as vital tools in this transformative landscape. As the aging population grows and chronic conditions become increasingly prevalent, traditional healthcare delivery methods face significant challenges, including accessibility and cost-effectiveness. By leveraging telehealth, patients are enabled to consult their healthcare providers from the comfort of their homes, leading to increased convenience and adherence to treatment plans. Remote monitoring systems utilize wearable devices and mobile applications to continuously track patients health metrics, allowing for proactive management of various health conditions. This shift not only empowers patients but also optimizes healthcare resources, demonstrating the potential of these technologies to improve the overall efficacy of healthcare delivery. As noted, Telehealth has the potential to revolutionize the way we deliver healthcare, especially for older adults and those with chronic conditions, underscoring the significant implications for longevity in health care. The integration of remote monitoring technologies holds promise for enhancing patient outcomes and reshaping care paradigms. By enabling healthcare providers to gather real-time data, remote monitoring facilitates timely interventions and reduces the need for hospital visits, ultimately contributing to better management of chronic diseases. The ability to analyze data from various sources allows for personalized treatment strategies, tailored to each patients unique circumstances. Additionally, this approach provides valuable insights into population health trends, contributing to a more comprehensive understanding of disease management and prevention. As researchers continue to explore the intersection of technology and healthcare, the findings will be crucial for informing policies and standards related to telehealth. By harnessing these capabilities, the healthcare system can move toward a more responsive and patient-centered model, making strides in the quest for longevity and quality of life throughout the aging process. The impact of telehealth and remote monitoring extends beyond individual health outcomes, influencing the broader dynamics of healthcare systems and society. As these technologies proliferate, they challenge traditional healthcare constructs, necessitating new frameworks of care delivery that prioritize accessibility and efficiency. In the context of a rapidly aging population, ensuring equitable access to telehealth services becomes paramount. Addressing disparities in technology access and digital literacy will be essential to fully realize the benefits of these innovations. As remote monitoring becomes commonplace, it has the potential to foster a sense of shared responsibility between patients and providers, leading to more engaged and informed healthcare consumers. With increasing reliance on telehealth, the paradigm of patient-provider interaction is evolving, paving the way for a future where longevity is not only attainable but sustainable. The question remains, however: are we prepared for the societal shifts these technologies will necessitate in our approach to health and longevity?

Robotics in Assisted Living

The integration of robotics into assisted living environments represents a transformative shift in how we approach care for the elderly and disabled. By deploying advanced robotic systems, we can enhance the quality of life for individuals who face mobility challenges or cognitive impairments. These robots, designed with user-friendly interfaces and empathetic interactions, provide companionship while also performing essential tasks such as medication reminders, mobility assistance, and emergency alerts. Such functionalities not only support the health and safety of residents but also alleviate the burden on caregivers, allowing them to focus on more complex emotional and social needs. The optimal deployment of robotics in these settings highlights the potential for technology to foster greater independence within vulnerable populations, aligning with broader goals of longevity and well-being that this essay explores. Crucially, the success of robotics in assisted living hinges on their ability to seamlessly integrate into existing care frameworks. Training for staff and residents alike on how to interact with these systems is essential for maximizing their benefits. Robotics should not replace human care but rather augment it, providing a hybrid model where technology and human compassion coexist. This approach can continually adapt through feedback loops, where data collected from both users and caregivers informs improvements in robot functionality. Images such as and effectively depict this multi-faceted integration by visualizing the interconnectedness of technology, biological feedback, and health outcomes, thereby emphasizing the systemic nature of care that robotics can enhance. These advancements suggest a promising future as we prepare for a society where longevity is a prominent reality. In addressing the ethical implications of robotics in assisted living, we must consider issues of autonomy, privacy, and human dignity. The use of intelligent systems raises questions about the potential for over-reliance on technology, potentially diminishing human interaction and relationships—a core tenet of caregiving. Ensuring that robotics are designed with ethical considerations in mind can mitigate these risks and enhance user acceptance. Ongoing discussions about the balance between technological intervention and human agency are critical. By incorporating images like and, which focus on health impacts and aging-related challenges, we can ground our analysis in visual data that illustrates the nuance necessary for ethical considerations. As we move towards a future of extended lifespans, it becomes imperative that our approaches to assisted living reflect not only the capabilities of technology but also the fundamental human needs it serves.

Year	Number of Robots Used	Nursing Homes using Robotics (%)	Average Cost per Robot
2020	15,000	25	30,000
2021	22,000	35	28,000
2022	35,000	45	27,000
2023	50,000	55	26,000

Robotics in Assisted Living Statistics

Smart Homes for Seniors

Advancements in smart home technology hold immense promise for enhancing the quality of life for seniors, particularly as longevity becomes increasingly feasible. By implementing integrated systems, elderly individuals can benefit from features designed to support independent living while addressing unique health needs. Smart sensors can monitor daily activities, detect falls, and even alert caregivers or emergency services when necessary. This proactive approach not only offers peace of mind but also enables older adults to maintain their autonomy. The automation of everyday tasks—such as adjusting lighting, controlling temperature, and managing appliances—further reduces the physical strain often associated with aging. Smart homes can create an environment where seniors feel safer and more empowered, thereby promoting a sense of belonging and well-being as they navigate the later stages of life. Integrating these technologies is essential to ensuring that aging populations can thrive in an increasingly digital world. The intersection of smart home technology and the aging population also raises important questions about accessibility and inclusivity. As seniors may have varying levels of tech-savviness, designing user-friendly interfaces remains crucial for widespread adoption. Older individuals often face challenges such as cognitive decline and reduced dexterity, which can hinder their ability to interact with complex systems. Addressing these barriers not only necessitates intuitive designs but also involves comprehensive education and training programs tailored to older adults. Encouraging familial support in this process can further facilitate successful integration. Family members can play a role in guiding their loved ones through the adoption of new technologies, ensuring they understand their capabilities and functionalities. Without a strong emphasis on accessibility, the potential benefits of smart homes could be undermined, limiting the positive impact of technological advancements on seniors' independence and overall quality of life. In addition to addressing practical concerns, the adoption of smart homes for seniors introduces important considerations regarding privacy and data security. As homes become filled with intelligent devices capable of collecting and transmitting sensitive information, seniors may be vulnerable to breaches of privacy. It is essential to implement stringent data protection measures to ensure that personal health information remains confidential and secure. Transparency in how data is collected, used, and shared is crucial for building trust between seniors and technology providers. In an era where personal data is increasingly commodified, care must be taken to prioritize ethical standards in the development of smart technologies for aging populations. Establishing policies that prioritize user consent and data security will ensure that as we continue to explore new possibilities for longevity, the well-being of the elder population remains at the forefront of technological innovation. By taking these considerations into account, we can pave the way for a future where smart homes enhance both the longevity and quality of life for seniors.

Year	Number of Smart Home Devices Used by Seniors	Percentage of Seniors Using Smart Homes	Improvement in Safety Features
2021	2,500,000	20	30% increase
2022	3,000,000	25	40% increase
2023	4,000,000	30	50% increase
2024	5,000,000	35	60% increase

Smart Homes for Seniors Statistics

XVII. THE FUTURE OF WORK IN AN AGING SOCIETY

As society forges ahead amidst increasing longevity, the workforce landscape is being reshaped in profound ways. With life expectancy extending well beyond traditional retirement age, organizations must adapt to accommodate a burgeoning demographic of older workers. These individuals come equipped with invaluable experience, wisdom, and resilience that can enhance productivity and mentorship within the workplace. As the workforce ages, there is a concurrent need to evolve job roles and expectations. Work environments must foster flexibility, accessibility, and inclusivity to harness the full potential of older employees while addressing challenges such as potential declines in physical health and the need for ongoing skill acquisition. Companies that effectively implement age-inclusive policies and training programs not only enhance employee satisfaction but also drive innovation by leveraging the diverse perspectives that come from a multi-generational workforce. Thus, addressing the needs of older workers is not merely an ethical obligation but a strategic business imperative. Simultaneously, advancements in technology are significantly impacting the future of work in an aging society. The ongoing integration of artificial intelligence, automation, and telecommuting tools provides exciting opportunities for older individuals to remain engaged and productive. As highlighted in images like, which depict how technology bridges gaps in health analysis and biomedicine, similar applications can be seen in workplace settings where tech assists in job performance. Remote work platforms enable older adults to contribute their expertise without the constraints of geographical limitations. Technologies facilitating lifelong learning, such as online education and virtual reality training, empower this demographic to continually adapt to new roles and industries. As these technological resources become more refined and accessible, they play a crucial role in reshaping work dynamics, ensuring that the talents of older generations are preserved and integrated into the evolving workforce. Emerging research emphasizes the importance of holistic approaches in creating a sustainable work environment within an aging society. Initiatives that focus on well-being, such as comprehensive health programs and supportive workplace cultures, are essential to maintaining a productive older workforce. The image, illustrating the interconnected mechanisms of biological aging and health determinants, serves as a reminder that employee health directly influences organizational performance. By investing in workplace wellness and creating supportive structures that encourage physical and mental health, companies can reduce absenteeism and enhance engagement among older employees. Fostering an inclusive environment that values lifelong contribution can inspire a generational collaboration, bridging gaps between younger and older employees. Such strategic measures not only enrich the organizational culture but also pave the way for a sustainable workforce that thrives on the combined strengths of individuals across all stages of life.

Year	Percentage of Population Over 65	Labor Force Participation Rate	Avg Age of Workers
2025	19.3	20.6	42
2030	21.6	22.4	43
2035	23.5	24.1	44
2040	25.9	25.8	45
2045	27.6	27.3	46

Future of Work in an Aging Society

Lifelong Learning and Employment

As society evolves towards a future where lifespans can extend significantly, the traditional landscape of employment must adapt in tandem. The adoption of emerging technologies and multidisciplinary knowledge, prominently identified in the health sciences through frameworks such as precision medicine, requires a workforce equipped with skills that transcend conventional educational trajectories. Lifelong learning becomes imperative for individuals aiming to thrive in dynamic work environments where continuous development of skills is essential. The rising importance of understanding complex biological aging mechanisms insinuates that professionals in healthcare, technology, and related fields must continuously engage in educational opportunities to stay relevant. This notion aligns with the visual mapping of interdisciplinary approaches from image, which illustrates biological processes impacting health and aging, showcasing the intricate relationships that professionals must navigate. Those who embrace lifelong learning are better positioned to adapt to these shifts, ensuring not only their employability but also their capacity to contribute to transformative advancements in their fields. The implications of extending lifespans raise critical questions about the sustainability of employment throughout an individual's life. As people live longer, they may pursue multiple careers or return to education later in life, challenging the notion of a linear career path. This shift necessitates revised corporate structures, promoting flexible work arrangements and continuous education programs that support employees at various life stages. Companies can encourage a culture of learning by providing resources for developing skills essential for navigating the healthcare landscape shaped by genetic editing and regenerative medicine, as discussed in image. As organizations recognize the value of an adaptable workforce, they foster resilience and innovation, thus maximizing productivity and job satisfaction. This holistic approach positions lifelong learning as fundamental not only for individual growth but also for economic sustainability, indicating a paradigm shift where learning is integrated into the very fabric of professional development. The role of societal attitudes toward education and employment will significantly shape the landscape of lifelong learning. As more people contemplate the longevity of their careers, cultural perceptions about aging and professional contribution will inevitably evolve. Societies must cultivate environments that celebrate continuous growth and adaptability, rather than stigmatizing age-related transitions in the workforce. Public and private sectors alike should collaborate to dismantle age biases, ensuring that programs addressing lifelong education and training are inclusive and accessible. Additionally, visual representations such as those in image elucidate the need for understanding the biological basis of aging, emphasizing the importance of informed policy-making in creating educational frameworks that support diverse populations. As communities embrace lifelong learning, they can tap into the full potential of their aging workforce, thereby fostering an inclusive economy prepared to meet the challenges and opportunities presented by extended lifespans.

Age Diversity in the Workplace

In increasingly diverse workplaces, the interplay between age and professional performance is becoming more pronounced. The inclusion of employees from various age groups not only enriches the work environment but also fosters a climate of innovation and creativity. When younger and older individuals collaborate, they bring together distinct perspectives shaped by differing life experiences and technological adaptiveness. This symbiosis has the potential to enhance problem-solving capabilities as diverse teams are more adept at generating a broader range of ideas. Leveraging the unique strengths of each age group can lead to more comprehensive decision-making processes, ultimately benefiting the organization as a whole. Such synergies highlight the importance of cultivating an inclusive culture that recognizes the contributions of all employees, regardless of their age. This diverse dynamic underscores both the economic and social implications of age diversity, necessitating strategic approaches from management to harness these benefits effectively. Addressing the challenges intertwined with age diversity is crucial for cultivating a thriving workplace. Age-related stereotypes often create barriers to collaboration, leading to potential conflicts and a lack of understanding among different age groups. Employers must actively combat these biases through targeted training programs that emphasize the value of age diversity, thereby preparing employees to appreciate varied contributions. Initiatives that encourage mentorship relationships or knowledge-sharing sessions can bolster intergenerational dialogue, allowing individuals to learn from each other's expertise and experiences. Additionally, companies must implement flexible policies that foster an accommodating environment for all employees. By facilitating adjustments in work schedules that consider the different needs of various age groups, organizations can minimize friction and build a cohesive workforce. Emphasizing these practices is essential for promoting a workplace culture that champions inclusivity while simultaneously harnessing the strengths of an age-diverse team. As discussions surrounding longevity continue to gain traction, the implications of an aging workforce become increasingly significant. The prospect of extended lifespans hints at a future where individuals may remain in the workforce longer than previous generations, reshaping traditional career trajectories. This shift could warrant a reevaluation of role definitions and workforce dynamics, paving the way for hybrid roles where younger and older individuals collaborate in unprecedented ways. As a result, organizations may find opportunities to harness the seasoned insights of older employees alongside the innovative ideas of younger personnel, ultimately leading to sustainable growth and productivity. To navigate this evolving landscape, businesses must reconsider their hiring practices, benefits, and training opportunities in light of an age-diverse workforce. As industries adapt to an aging population, the potential benefits of fostering age diversity in the workplace are profound, paving the way for a future where experience and innovation coexist harmoniously. Supporting this discussion, the image offers a valuable visual representation of the complex interactions among biological aging processes. Not only does it map out various mechanisms affecting aging, but it also underscores the relevance of understanding these biological factors in the context of workplace dynamics as longevity trends rise. By integrating such visual tools into the analysis, the exploration of age diversity can become more nuanced, enriching the conversations around the future of work in the context of extended lifespans.

Adapting Work Environments for Older Adults

As the workforce ages, organizations must reconsider traditional work environments to accommodate the unique needs of older adults. This adaptation extends beyond mere ergonomic adjustments; it encompasses a holistic approach that embraces psychological and social dimensions. Flexible working hours and the option for remote work can significantly enhance productivity and job satisfaction for older employees, allowing them to balance personal health needs with professional responsibilities. Fostering an inclusive culture that values the contributions and experiences of older adults can effectively mitigate ageism, creating a more cohesive workplace. Such cultural shifts not only benefit aging workers but also enrich the organization as a whole, ensuring a diverse array of perspectives that can drive innovation and problem-solving. Integrating these strategies creates a foundation for a supportive environment where older adults can thrive, thus maximizing both their work potential and overall quality of life. Equally vital is the integration of technology within work environments to facilitate the adaptability of older adults. As workplaces increasingly rely on digital tools, ensuring accessibility is paramount. Implementing user-friendly software that accommodates varying levels of technological proficiency can empower older workers to engage fully with their tasks. Additionally, the inclusion of assistive technologies, such as speech recognition and screen magnification software, can help mitigate the challenges older employees may face. Training programs tailored specifically for older individuals can further bridge the technology gap, enhancing their comfort and competence in navigating digital workplaces. Collectively, these efforts can help dismantle barriers and foster a work culture that not only supports but also leverages the strengths of older adults. By embracing technology as an enabler, organizations can create environments that promote collaboration across age groups and enhance overall workplace productivity. The imperative to adapt work environments for older adults aligns with broader societal shifts towards longevity and quality of life. The prospect of living to 150 years necessitates rethinking not just individual health strategies, but also how work roles contribute to an enriching later life. With increasing longevity, work can no longer be viewed merely as a means of financial support; instead, it should be embraced as a crucial element of identity and social engagement for older adults. By prioritizing meaningful work experiences, organizations can help ensure that older employees find purpose in their roles, leading to improved mental and emotional well-being. This paradigm shift highlights the need for interdisciplinary research and collaboration across fields such as psychology, occupational therapy, and gerontology to craft work environments that cater specifically to the aging population. In doing so, society can enhance the potential for thriving human experiences well into later years, fostering a richer tapestry of life as we navigate the implications of extended lifespans.

XVIII. LONGEVITY AND GLOBAL HEALTH

As societies grapple with the increasing longevity of their populations, the imperative to create robust healthcare systems becomes paramount. Many nations are witnessing a demographic shift, with an expanding proportion of elderly individuals who require medical attention, chronic disease management, and supportive services. This trend brings to the forefront the role of integrated health plans that prioritize preventive care and early intervention. Investing in health-related technology, as visualized in, can enhance the capability to predict health outcomes and facilitate personalized medicine. Such advancements promise to transform how health is managed across the lifespan, ultimately contributing to improved quality of life in older age. While technology offers unprecedented opportunities, the challenge remains to ensure equitable access to these innovations so that all populations can reap the benefits. Thus, a focus on inclusivity in health services becomes essential in promoting longevity as a global health objective. The intersection of culture, economic conditions, and public policy in shaping the aging experience cannot be overlooked. Different societies have varied beliefs and practices regarding aging, which significantly impact both mental and physical health outcomes. In cultures that honor the elderly, there is often a more significant emphasis on community support and social engagement, contributing to better psychological well-being and overall health. A study presented in reveals that mental health interventions focusing on social connectivity can enhance longevity outcomes, suggesting that integrating mental health awareness into traditional healthcare approaches is crucial. Bridging the gap among diverse cultural perspectives on aging fosters an environment where innovative practices can flourish, aiding in the creation of more effective health policies. In this context, embracing cultural sensitivity becomes critical in shaping health initiatives aimed at enhancing life expectancy across global populations. The global implications of increasing longevity extend far beyond individual health; they pose complex challenges and opportunities for economies and societies at large. As life expectancy rises, the workforce dynamics and economic productivity are bound to shift, creating a need for adaptive strategies that address the aging populace. The economic landscape could benefit greatly from a focus on lifelong learning and skills development, ensuring that older adults can remain active contributors to society. Evidence from studies showcased in demonstrates economic models that emphasize intergenerational collaboration and supportive work environments, which can lead to more sustainable economies. This complex balancing act will require forward-thinking regulations and policies that attain a societal consensus on the value of extending longevity. By fostering discussions around the economic ramifications of longevity, societies can align their priorities with the future horizon of health and well-being, setting a solid foundation for successful intergenerational coexistence.

Health Disparities and Longevity

Racial and socioeconomic factors play a pivotal role in determining health outcomes and longevity, illustrating the pervasive nature of health disparities in modern society. Minority populations often experience higher rates of chronic diseases like diabetes and hypertension due to limited access to healthcare, nutritional foods, and safe living environments. A glaring example is the impact of systemic inequalities, which can lead to a significant discrepancy in life expectancy between affluent and marginalized communities. The complex interplay of social determinants—including education, income, and neighborhood conditions—contributes to these disparities, compounding existing health challenges. This underscores the necessity for targeted public health interventions that address underlying social injustices, ultimately striving for equitable health access to ameliorate the longevity gap. Evidence-based strategies, such as community engagement and health education, can empower vulnerable populations and contribute to mitigating these disparities, indicating a clear pathway toward improved longevity for underrepresented groups. The concept of biological aging further complicates the discussion of health disparities, as individuals from different backgrounds may exhibit varying aging patterns influenced by genetic, environmental, and behavioral factors. Emerging research indicates that certain epigenetic markers, identified through methods such as Methylation Profile Scores (MPSs), reflect biological age more accurately than chronological age, suggesting a need for tailored healthcare approaches. By understanding the mechanisms of biological aging, particularly among diverse populations, health professionals can develop more precise interventions that address specific vulnerabilities associated with accelerated aging. Individuals suffering from chronic stress due to socioeconomic factors might experience quicker biological aging, prompting a review of healthcare accessibility and prevention strategies. Consequently, integrating biological insights into public health frameworks can lead to meaningful improvements in health outcomes and longevity, as practitioners adopt a more personalized and inclusive approach to health management. This nuanced understanding of the biological underpinnings of aging underscores the need to consider diverse experiences in health policy and practice. Advancements in biotechnology and regenerative medicine present both opportunities and challenges in addressing health disparities and promoting longevity. Innovations such as genetic editing and cellular therapies hold the potential to revolutionize treatment for chronic diseases, often prevalent in underserved populations. The accessibility of these groundbreaking technologies remains a concern, as disparities in healthcare resources could widen the longevity gap rather than close it. Ensuring equitable access to these advancements requires comprehensive policy frameworks that prioritize inclusivity and affordability. Ethical considerations surrounding gene editing and biotechnological interventions necessitate public discourse and community involvement to avoid exacerbating existing inequalities. By actively engaging stakeholders from various demographics, policymakers can design strategies that leverage technological advancements to foster a healthier, more equitable society. In this light, the pursuit of longevity must go hand in hand with efforts to dismantle barriers to healthcare access, promoting a future where advancements benefit all segments of the population, rather than a select few. In this context, serves as a critical visual representation of the interconnections between health disparities and biological aging, reinforcing the arguments presented in the paragraphs. The depiction of various aging clocks through a multi-omic lens is particularly relevant as it highlights how different dimensions of health can influence aging processes, emphasizing the importance of inclusivity in research and policy-making. By integrating such imagery, the analysis gains depth and clarity, illustrating the urgency for an approach that acknowledges the complexities of health disparities as it pertains to longevity.

Group	Life Expectancy (Years)	Premature Mortality Rate (per 100,000)	Chronic Disease Prevalence (%)
White Non-Hispanic	78.8	170	55
Black Non-Hispanic	74.7	230	60
Hispanic	81.8	140	50
Asian American	86.5	100	40
Native American	75.3	250	65

Health Disparities and Their Impact on Longevity

Global Aging Trends

Demographic shifts are altering the global landscape in unprecedented ways, as populations age at an accelerated rate. According to the United Nations, the proportion of people aged 60 years or older is expected to double from about 12% to 22% of the global population by 2050. This dramatic increase poses significant challenges and opportunities for societies worldwide. Aging populations may strain healthcare systems, requiring increased resources for geriatric care and chronic disease management. There is a growing need for policies that promote active aging and enable older individuals to contribute meaningfully to society. These trends necessitate a paradigm shift in how we perceive aging—not merely as a period of decline but as an opportunity for continued growth, engagement, and productivity. Addressing these demographic changes involves not only medical advancements but also social innovations that foster intergenerational collaboration and support mechanisms, integral aspects of a society grappling with its aging population. Chronic diseases, often prevalent in older populations, underscore the importance of innovations in biotechnology and regenerative medicine as fundamental responses to global aging trends. Advances in our understanding of aging biology have paved the way for breakthroughs like gene therapy and stem cell treatments that promise to mitigate age-related ailments. Research indicates that targeted therapies may enhance health spans, allowing individuals to experience longer periods of vitality and well-being. The integration of precision medicine into treatment plans can tailor interventions to specific genetic and environmental factors, enhancing their efficacy. While such technologies hold great potential, their implementation raises ethical considerations about accessibility and equity in healthcare. Ensuring that these advancements are available to all demographic segments, especially underserved populations, is critical for creating an inclusive approach to longevity that benefits society as a whole. Culturally varied perspectives on aging significantly influence societal readiness to embrace longer lifespans. In some cultures, elderly individuals are revered for their wisdom and contributions, resulting in programs that actively engage them in community life. Conversely, in societies that prioritize youth, aging is often stigmatized, leading to a neglect of older adults needs and experiences. This dichotomy shapes policy responses and social structures, affecting how communities adapt to demographic changes. As nations grapple with increasing longevity, they must consider these cultural frameworks and their implications for social cohesion and intergenerational relationships. Future approaches to longevity must promote inclusivity and respect for diverse age-related experiences while fostering environments where all members of society—regardless of age—can thrive. Such cultural awareness can inform more effective strategies in addressing the multifaceted challenges posed by global aging trends.

Year	Global Population Aged 65+	Total Population (%)
2020	727,000,000	9.3
2025	850,000,000	10.4
2030	1,000,000,000	12.2
2035	1,200,000,000	14.5
2040	1,400,000,000	16.5
2045	1,600,000,000	18.7
2050	1,800,000,000	20.7

Global Aging Trends Data

International Collaboration in Aging Research

Collaborative international efforts in aging research are paramount for addressing the multifaceted challenges posed by an increasingly aging global population. As countries face unique health demographics influenced by cultural, economic, and environmental factors, pooling resources and knowledge can facilitate innovative solutions. Researchers from diverse geographic regions can work together to analyze large datasets, thereby generating insights that are difficult to achieve in isolation. This collaboration permits the exploration of global phenomena, such as shared health problems among aging populations and effective interventions tailored to different societal contexts. Establishing robust partnerships can strengthen the research infrastructure, leading to cross-pollination of ideas, methodologies, and technologies that drive breakthroughs in the understanding of biological aging and its implications. The integration of technology and a systems biology approach undoubtedly benefits from international collaboration, particularly as researchers are increasingly accessing and sharing vast databases. The migration towards a more interconnected scientific community emphasizes the importance of adopting a multi-omic perspective in aging research. This involves the convergence of various disciplines such as genomics, proteomics, and microbiomics to understand aging on a fundamental level. In pooling these distinct but complementary academic fields, researchers can create refined aging clocks that better assess biological age and health trajectories across diverse populations. The prospect of developing personalized healthcare systems hinges upon these collaborative efforts, with potential implications for precision medicine in gerontology that can cater to specific demands arising from aging demographics worldwide. This synergy can ultimately enhance the health span—the period of life spent in good health—of aging individuals while addressing disparities inherent in global health systems. The ethical considerations surrounding aging research are significantly enriched through international dialogue and cooperation. Different cultural attitudes toward aging and longevity can influence the policies and practices adopted in various jurisdictions. Engaging in discussions with global partners can foreground these values, ensuring that emerging technologies and therapeutic interventions remain ethically sound and culturally sensitive. Consequently, addressing concerns such as equity in access to longevity-enhancing treatments, consideration for the aging workforce, and appropriate mental health strategies becomes a collaborative endeavor that transcends borders. A unified international approach can lead to the formulation of comprehensive frameworks that protect individual well-being while also honoring global diversity in experiencing aging. This collaborative ethos strengthens the field, potentially paving the way for a more sustainable and ethically aligned future in the quest for extending human longevity.

XIX. PSYCHOLOGICAL ADAPTATION TO LONGEVITY

As humanity approaches the potential for extended lifespans, adapting psychologically to longevity becomes an essential consideration. The mental adjustment required to embrace significantly lengthened life spans may provoke both opportunities and challenges. Individuals must develop resilience to navigate the complexities of aging, including health declines and the loss of loved ones, while also seizing the chance to pursue long-held dreams and ambitions. This duality can lead to a rich tapestry of experiences, but also the risk of existential anxiety and depression as individuals grapple with the notion of prolonged life. The transformative health paradigms emerging from fields such as regenerative medicine and genetic engineering, as outlined in, support the need for a nuanced understanding of how psychological well-being impacts quality of life as we age. Thus, the interplay of hope and apprehension in the context of longevity highlights the importance of mental adaptation strategies for successful aging. The perception of aging is largely shaped by cultural narratives and societal frameworks, both of which must evolve in light of potential life extension. Traditionally, many cultures view aging through a lens of decline and loss, often neglecting the opportunities that prolonged life can present. To construct a beneficial approach to longevity, psychological adaptation requires not just individual growth but also a collective shift in perspectives about what it means to age. Societal acceptance of advanced healthcare practices, like those depicted in, can enhance community awareness and support networks, ultimately fostering positive attitudes toward aging.

Emphasizing the value of lifelong learning, intergenerational connections, and active community participation can contribute to a vibrant experience of old age. By reshaping these cultural narratives, society can create an environment that not only anticipates longer lives but celebrates the richness these additional years can bring. Psychological adaptation to longevity necessitates rethinking traditional roles and life stages in family and professional contexts. The rise in life expectancy may require individuals to reassess aspirations and expectations related to career progression, family structures, and personal goals. As evidenced in, the cumulative wisdom and experience that comes with extended lifespans can equip individuals to make meaningful contributions to society at various life stages. This shift also poses challenges, such as the possibility of intergenerational conflict and the strain on resources. Individuals and families will benefit from proactive planning for future life stages, balancing aspirations with realistic assessments of physical and mental health. Addressing psychological readiness to embrace these changes is critical to leverage the potential benefits of longevity fully, ensuring that additional years translate into enhanced well-being and fulfillment rather than burden and distress.

Coping with Extended Lifespan

The prospect of extended lifespans raises significant considerations about the coping mechanisms required for individuals and societies alike. As medical advancements increase the feasibility of living beyond 100 years, attention must turn to the psychological and emotional challenges that accompany prolonged life. Mental health, often overlooked in discussions about longevity, becomes a paramount concern. Individuals may face issues such as loneliness, cognitive decline, and decreased motivation, making mental wellness strategies essential. Innovative interventions, like those seen in the potential applications of deep generative reinforcement learning in mental health analysis, can play a crucial role in this context. By understanding patterns in behavior and offering tailored support, these technologies help mitigate the effects of isolation and mental deterioration among the elderly. The intertwining of aging with mental health care signifies a critical intersection that must be prioritized in preparing for extended lifespans, ensuring quality of life alongside increased longevity. Physical health also requires a comprehensive approach to effectively cope with extended lifespans. Growing evidence suggests that integrating nutrition, exercise, and preventive healthcare is vital in managing the aging process. As illustrated in the comparative studies of various dietary approaches, such as the ketogenic and Mediterranean diets, a holistic view of nutrition must be embraced to aid not just longevity but also functional aging. These diets have shown promise in enhancing cognitive functions and reducing physiological risks, thereby promoting a healthier, longer life. Additionally, advancements in biomarkers, as presented in the multi-omic frameworks for aging, allow for more personalized healthcare strategies. By understanding individual biological profiles, tailored interventions can be crafted to address specific health risks, empowering individuals to take charge of their longevity proactively. The convergence of nutrition, physical activity, and personalized medicine represents an essential strategy for coping with the realities of extended lifespans. Social structures and cultural attitudes are equally critical in navigating the implications of longer lives. The potential for extended lifespans necessitates a reevaluation of familial and societal roles, particularly regarding caregiving and intergenerational relationships. Evolving family dynamics might lead to increased responsibilities on younger generations, who may be required to support aging relatives for longer periods. This shift necessitates societal support systems that cater to both younger and older populations, promoting inclusivity and mutual understanding. Cultural perceptions of aging play a significant role in how societies adapt to longevity. Countries with progressive views on aging often create environments that celebrate elder contributions, fostering respect and engagement rather than isolation. As seen in various global practices addressing aging, cultivating positive cultural narratives surrounding older adults can enhance intergenerational exchanges and encourage environments where wisdom is valued. Thus, preparing for a demographic shift towards older populations involves not only healthcare and individual strategies but also a fundamental transformation in societal attitudes and structures.

Identity and Self-Perception in Old Age

As individuals transition into old age, self-perception often undergoes profound transformations influenced by both internal and external factors. One's identity, composed of accumulated experiences, relationships, and societal roles, can become more pronounced or questioned during this phase. In many cases, older adults reflect on their life's achievements, grappling with the meaning ascribed to those experiences. This introspection can elicit feelings of fulfillment or regret, shaping their self-image. Factors such as societal expectations, historical context, and cultural attitudes toward aging play pivotal roles in how the elderly view themselves. Those in cultures that revere the wisdom of elders may experience a heightened sense of purpose and self-worth. This interplay between personal reflection and external societal norms highlights the complexity of identity and self-perception in later life, suggesting that perspectives on aging can profoundly influence psychological well-being and quality of life. Changes in physical appearance and health status can significantly impact self-esteem and self-worth for older adults, often leading to an evolving sense of identity. As bodies alter due to aging processes or health conditions, the internal narrative may shift from one emphasizing vitality to one that grapples with limitations. This deterioration can lead individuals to question their previous roles and how they view their capabilities. Specifically, as discussed in the frameworks of biological aging and the mechanisms influencing resilience, such as the findings from image, these alterations challenge both personal identity and societal expectations. The adaptation to these changes often necessitates a redefinition of self-concept; individuals may have to embrace new roles or priorities that highlight emotional connections and intellectual capabilities rather than physical appearance. Thus, the changing realities of aging necessitate a sophisticated balancing act between maintaining an established identity and adapting to new life circumstances. Emerging technologies and societal shifts related to longevity further complicate identity and self-perception in old age. As advancements in biotechnology and regenerative medicine pave pathways toward extended life, this potential for longevity can provoke a reassessment of what it means to age. With possibilities of enhanced health and extended vitality, older adults may find themselves reimagining their roles within family and society. While image highlights the potential for deep generative reinforcement learning to enhance mental health and well-being, this suggests a future where older adults can actively participate in various societal spheres, thus redefining their identities as contributors rather than dependent figures. This evolution prompts significant philosophical inquiries about purpose and fulfillment in extended old age, encouraging an exploration of personal aspirations that transcend traditional age-related limitations. Consequently, the interplay of technological advancements and shifting societal perceptions presents a fundamental opportunity for older generations to cultivate a renewed and dynamic sense of identity in an era characterized by extended life expectancy.

Resilience and Aging

Resilience in the aging process is increasingly recognized as a key factor in enhancing the quality of life among older adults. As individuals navigate the physical and cognitive challenges associated with aging, their capacity to adapt, recover, and thrive significantly influences their overall health and longevity. Research has shown that resilience is not merely a personal trait but is intricately linked to social support, environmental factors, and a sense of purpose. Communities that foster strong social networks tend to promote resilience, leading to enhanced well-being and reduced susceptibility to age-related conditions. This interconnectedness is highlighted in imagery that showcases the systems approach to biological and health dynamics, as seen in.

Such frameworks suggest that resilience is cultivated not just within the individual, but through supportive relationships and community structures that encourage healthy behaviors and emotional strength, ultimately allowing older adults to face the challenges of extended longevity with greater fortitude. The implications of resilience extend beyond personal health; they encompass the societal dimensions of aging as well. As life expectancy increases, the cumulative effects of stress and adversity can manifest in greater public health challenges. Older adults who exhibit high levels of resilience can mitigate these risks, but the necessary resources and support systems must be in place. Programs aimed at fostering resilience—whether they encompass mental health interventions, physical activity initiatives, or community engagement opportunities—can play a decisive role in shaping health outcomes for an aging population. Engaging in preventive measures and promoting lifelong learning experiences can significantly enhance cognitive function and emotional adaptability. The holistic approach represented in speaks to the necessity of integrating these diverse factors in health planning, as nurturing resilience not only enhances individual lives but also contributes to the sustainability of health care systems as they adapt to a growing older demographic. In considering the future of longevity, the role of resilience in aging cannot be overstated. As we explore the potential for living to an advanced age—perhaps even reaching 150 years—it becomes essential to cultivate a framework that prioritizes psychological health and adaptability. Within this context, it is paramount to recognize that resilience is a skill, one that can be cultivated through conscious effort and community support. The challenges associated with a longer life, including chronic illness and mental decline, underscore the necessity for resilience training and resources that equip individuals to confront these obstacles effectively. As such, it is crucial to align societal strategies with the understanding that it is not the physical challenges that set you back, it is the mental. *"It is not the physical challenges that set you back, it is the mental. You have to summon the will to keep going, step after step, day after day."* (Dr. Rick Nielsen). By fostering resilience in aging populations, we can not only enhance individual health outcomes but also ensure that society is prepared to embrace the opportunities and challenges presented by unprecedented longevity. The intersection of resilience and aging thus emerges as a vital area of focus for researchers, policymakers, and communities alike.

Age Group	Average Resilience Score	Percentage With Resilience Skills	Source
60-69	7.2	65	National Institute on Aging (2022)
70-79	6.9	62	National Institute on Aging (2022)
80-89	6.5	58	National Institute on Aging (2022)
90+	5.8	50	National Institute on Aging (2022)

Aging and Resilience Data

XX. THE ROLE OF COMMUNITY IN LONGEVITY

The social fabric of communities plays a crucial role in fostering environments conducive to longevity. Individuals who belong to strong social networks often experience better health outcomes than those who are isolated. This phenomenon can be attributed to the emotional and practical support communities provide, which are essential in mitigating stress and promoting well-being. Engagement in communal activities not only offers a sense of belonging but also encourages healthier lifestyle choices, such as exercise and balanced nutrition. Studies suggest that communal eating and shared physical activities enhance adherence to healthful behaviors, ultimately impacting longevity positively. A relevant example of this dynamic can be seen in the communities discussed in Part (a) of, where interconnected areas such as precision medicine and mental health analysis underscore the importance of community in supporting individual health trajectories. By fostering supportive environments, communities can play a pivotal role in enhancing quality of life and extending life spans. Intentional communities, particularly those structured around communal living and shared values, can significantly influence longevity through their focus on social cohesion and mutual aid. Many cultures emphasize the importance of familial and communal ties, which function as safety nets during life's challenges. These networks can motivate individuals to engage in preventive health practices and attend regular health check-ups, given the collective responsibility often present in such setups. The Mediterranean diet and lifestyle, highlighted in, reflects not only dietary choices but also the communal aspects of eating and socializing, which contribute to improved health outcomes. Research indicates that individuals within tightly-knit communities often enjoy lower rates of chronic diseases, suggesting that the collaborative and supportive nature of these environments fosters resilience and promotes healthier living. By nurturing interdependence and social responsibility, communities become significant agents in the quest for longevity. Emphasizing the role of community in the discourse of longevity also invites considerations of inclusivity and access to resources. Communities that prioritize health equity by ensuring all members have access to healthcare, nutritional resources, and education tend to cultivate healthier populations. Research outlined in Part (b) of reveals that when health interventions are community-focused and culturally competent, they yield higher engagement and better outcomes. This inclusivity also extends to integrating perspectives from various disciplines, such as healthcare, psychology, and community planning. Recognizing the interplay between environmental factors and health elucidates why community-oriented approaches are essential. The systemic barriers faced by marginalized populations demonstrate that without proactive community engagement and support, the potential benefits of advancements in longevity could exacerbate existing inequalities. Acknowledging and fostering communities that are equitable and nurturing is imperative in shaping a future where longevity becomes a realistic possibility for all.

Social Engagement and Longevity

The intricate interplay between social engagement and longevity has gained considerable attention in recent gerontological research. Evidence suggests that individuals who maintain strong social connections tend to experience enhanced well-being and increased lifespan. These connections can manifest through relationships with family, friendships, and community involvement, which serve as critical buffers against stress and health declines associated with aging. Studies show that loneliness and social isolation are significant predictors of mortality, often comparable to the risks posed by smoking or obesity. Engaging with others promotes cognitive function, emotional resilience, and physical activity, all of which are essential factors in sustaining health as one ages. Social networks often facilitate access to resources and support that can directly impact health outcomes, such as assistance in navigating healthcare needs or engaging in health-promoting activities. This underscores the notion that social engagement not only enriches life quality but also holds profound implications for longevity. Cultural perceptions of social engagement also play a pivotal role in shaping longevity outcomes. Different societies embody unique norms regarding familial obligations, community participation, and social behaviors, which influence how individuals engage with their social circles. In cultures where community and familial ties are prioritized, individuals may experience strengthened support systems that contribute to healthier aging. In Mediterranean cultures characterized by strong family bonds and communal activities, older adults are often found to exhibit lower incidence rates of chronic illnesses and improved overall well-being. This suggests that integrating cultural values into health promotion strategies could be beneficial in fostering a sense of belonging and purpose among older adults. By embracing the diverse ways in which societies foster social connections, health interventions can be tailored more effectively, ultimately enhancing longevity and creating healthier communities. Incorporating technology into the realm of social engagement presents both opportunities and challenges. With the rise of digital platforms, social connectivity has expanded beyond geographical limitations, empowering older adults to maintain relationships and engage with their communities. Reliance on technology can also perpetuate feelings of isolation if it replaces face-to-face interactions. Disparities in digital literacy and access can exacerbate existing inequalities among older populations, potentially widening the gap in longevity outcomes. Balancing the benefits of technological advancements with traditional forms of social engagement is crucial. Fostering environments that encourage in-person socialization, while also leveraging technology to enhance connectivity, could lead to a more comprehensive approach in promoting longevity. Understanding how these dynamics interact is vital as we explore the future of aging in a society increasingly influenced by technological change. Through a multifaceted approach, we can better position ourselves to support individuals in achieving not only longer lives but also richer, more fulfilling experiences.

Community Resources for Seniors

The foundation of community resources for seniors is essential for fostering healthy aging and enhancing the quality of life among older adults. These resources encompass a variety of services such as healthcare access, nutritional support, and social activities, which are crucial as individuals seek to navigate the complexities of prolonged longevity. With advances in fields such as biotechnology and regenerative medicine, there exists a distinct opportunity to harness these community offerings to support not only physical health but also mental and emotional well-being. Programs that promote social engagement and intergenerational interaction, for instance, can significantly mitigate feelings of loneliness and isolation, common among seniors. Thus, community organizations play a vital role in creating supportive networks that can translate advancements in healthcare into practical, everyday support for the elderly, aligning with the upcoming shifts toward an elongated lifespan. Access to comprehensive healthcare resources within the community is vital for seniors, especially as advancements in medical technology enhance lifespan. Services such as telehealth consultations enable seniors to receive necessary care without the burdensome travel often associated with traditional visits. Local health departments and nonprofit organizations frequently provide educational workshops on disease prevention and management tailored to older adults. This proactive approach can lead to improved health outcomes by empowering seniors with knowledge about their conditions and the means to manage them effectively. Collaborative efforts between healthcare providers and community organizations can ensure that these resources are not only accessible but also tailored to meet the diverse needs of an aging population. The integration of technology into these services, as discussed in various contemporary health frameworks, enhances their effectiveness and outreach, illustrating the potential of community resources to adapt in the face of an aging society. The implications of community resources extend beyond individual health, impacting local economies and societal structures as a whole. Investing in programs that support aging populations helps to alleviate burdens on healthcare systems by promoting preventive care and healthy lifestyles. These initiatives can cultivate a positive community ethos, encouraging younger generations to value and engage with their elders. In an era where the prospect of living significantly longer is becoming more plausible, communities that prioritize resources for seniors will not only enhance the lives of older citizens but will also cultivate a more inclusive and supportive society overall. By fostering environments where seniors feel valued and connected, communities can harness the power of collective experience and wisdom, ultimately enriching the fabric of society as a whole. The synergy between aging populations and community resources represents a critical element in ensuring a thriving future for all generations, thereby reinforcing the need for continuous investment in these vital programs. Image references such as reinforce the notion of interconnectedness among various factors influencing senior health. The comprehensive nature of community resource systems, depicted in Visions of Health, exemplifies how deep learning methodologies can enhance understanding and implementation of innovative health solutions for seniors.

City	Senior Centers	Home Health Aides	Meals on Wheels Programs	Senior Housing Facilities	Adult Day Care Centers
New York City	250	15,600	10	221	50
Los Angeles	180	13,000	15	180	40
Chicago	120	90,00	8	150	35
Houston	100	8,500	12	120	30
Phoenix	90	7,000	9	110	25

Community Resources for Seniors

Volunteerism and Its Benefits

Engaging in volunteerism serves as a pivotal mechanism for fostering community building and social cohesion. As individuals dedicate their time to causes that resonate with them, they create connections that transcend socio-economic barriers, promoting a sense of belonging and unity. Volunteer activities, whether in local shelters or global initiatives, allow individuals to collaborate with diverse groups, offering a rich tapestry of experiences that enhance personal growth and understanding. This is crucial as society moves toward a future where longer lifespans may alter traditional community structures and interpersonal relationships. By cultivating a sense of togetherness through shared goals, volunteer efforts can mitigate feelings of isolation that often accompany aging. An emphasis on volunteerism not only enriches the lives of those directly involved but also contributes to a resilient social fabric that can better support individuals living longer lives. The synergy created by such communal engagements lays the groundwork for healthier, more sustained social interactions. The personal benefits of volunteerism extend beyond mere altruism and into tangible psychological and physical health improvements. Engaging in volunteer work has been linked to higher levels of happiness and life satisfaction, with studies showing that individuals who volunteer report lower rates of depression and anxiety. This correlation aligns with emerging research that connects active community participation with longer life expectancy, suggesting that helping others may indeed help volunteers themselves. As the exploration of longevity advances—driven by scientific innovations such as biotechnology and regenerative medicine—incorporating volunteerism into lifestyle choices could enhance holistic well-being. The act of giving regularly prompts volunteers to maintain social contacts and cultivate a support network, which is essential as individuals age and potentially face increasing health challenges. Thus, volunteerism merits consideration as a viable strategy for promoting not only community welfare but also personal health over extended lifespans, ensuring that the journey toward longevity is a fulfilling one. Looking ahead, the role of volunteerism will likely become more vital as societies adapt to the new realities of extended life expectancy. Communities may need to shift their perception of aging, recognizing the potential for older adults to contribute actively and meaningfully through volunteer initiatives. This reimagining of aging challenges stereotypes that depict older individuals solely as receivers of care rather than as valuable community assets. By nurturing a culture of volunteerism, societies can leverage the skills and wisdom of older generations, transforming perceptions of aging into opportunities for lifelong engagement. Future frameworks exploring longevity should include volunteerism as a core component, promoting opportunities for intergenerational collaboration that benefit both younger and older populations alike. Such initiatives will not only address the emotional and psychological aspects of aging but also reinforce the interdependence required for sustained community health in an era of unprecedented longevity.

Age Group	Benefits Reported (%)	Community Impact Score
18-24	82	75
25-34	79	80
35-44	77	85
45-54	74	88
55-64	71	90
65+	68	92

Volunteerism Benefits by Age Group

XXI. INNOVATIONS IN PALLIATIVE CARE

As advancements in medical science pave the way for longer lifespans, palliative care is experiencing significant innovations that enhance the quality of life for patients facing serious illnesses. One notable development is the integration of technology into palliative care practices. Telehealth platforms are now being employed to provide remote consultations, allowing patients to access specialized care from their homes. This approach not only broadens the reach of palliative care services but also empowers individuals to maintain connections with healthcare providers regardless of geographical limitations. The use of data analytics has enabled palliative care teams to better understand patient needs and tailor interventions accordingly. This data-driven approach fosters a more personalized care experience, aligning treatment options with individual preferences and values, which is paramount in end-of-life discussions. Such technological innovations indicate a transformative shift in palliative care that emphasizes accessibility and patient-centeredness, facilitating a more dignified approach to serious illness. Empathy-driven interventions are another critical innovation enriching palliative care. The growing recognition of the psychological and emotional dimensions of serious illness has led to the incorporation of holistic practices that consider the comprehensive well-being of patients. This includes integrating mental health professionals into the palliative care team to address anxiety, depression, and other psychological burdens that patients may face. Additionally, support systems such as patient and family counseling, and community resources are increasingly being woven into care plans. By fostering open communication and providing emotional support, these initiatives create an environment where patients feel valued and understood. Research indicates that such interventions not only enhance patients overall satisfaction with care but also contribute to improved health outcomes. This holistic approach signifies a paradigm shift in how palliative care is perceived and delivered, emphasizing the importance of emotional support as a cornerstone of quality care. Cultural competency has emerged as a vital component of innovative palliative care, recognizing the diverse values and beliefs that influence patient experiences and treatment decisions. As society evolves toward a more multicultural landscape, palliative care providers are increasingly trained to understand cultural sensitivities and incorporate them into care plans. This includes respecting patients' religious beliefs, family dynamics, and cultural practices that may affect end-of-life decisions. Some cultures may prioritize family involvement in decision-making processes, while others may hold different views on the desirability of aggressive interventions. The acknowledgment of these cultural factors empowers patients and families, ensuring that care aligns with their values and preferences. As openness to diverse cultural perspectives grows, it contributes to more equitable palliative care practices, ultimately leading to enhanced patient satisfaction and outcomes. This emphasis on cultural competency represents a crucial step toward making palliative care more responsive to the needs of an increasingly diverse population, ensuring that all individuals facing serious illness receive care that resonates with their unique backgrounds.

Year	Innovation	Impact
2020	Telehealth Services	Increased accessibility to palliative care services by 50%
2021	Integrated Care Models	Reduction in hospital readmissions by 30%
2022	Artificial Intelligence Tools	Improved patient outcome prediction accuracy by 40%
2023	Patient-Centered Care Programs	Enhanced patient satisfaction scores by 25%

Palliative Care Innovations Statistics

Importance of End-of-Life Care

The process of aging inevitably leads to a myriad of health challenges that warrant comprehensive planning for care during the end-of-life phase. In this context, end-of-life care is crucial not only for ensuring that individuals receive compassionate and appropriate treatment but also for supporting their families during a profoundly difficult time. Care approaches, which may include hospice and palliative services, aim to address physical, emotional, and spiritual needs, making it imperative for health care systems to prioritize these services. While scientific advancements can prolong life, they also complicate the process of dying, often leading to a protracted decline that can diminish quality of life. As we explore the possibility of living well into our 150s, the challenge will not only be about extending life but also about refining the end-of-life experience in a way that respects individual desires and dignity. Hence, understanding the importance of end-of-life care becomes essential for informed discussions about longevity and quality of life. Expanding the focus to societal implications, it is clear that effective end-of-life care can have far-reaching effects on health care systems and public policy. Integrating comprehensive palliative care into routine health care can reduce the overall burden on hospitals and emergency services by minimizing unnecessary interventions during the terminal phase. Training health care providers to recognize and respect the values and preferences of dying patients allows for a more humane approach to care. This humanization is paramount, especially when faced with the ethical dilemmas surrounding advancements in biotechnology that may prolong life but do not necessarily enhance the quality of those extended years. Research in end-of-life care, including advancements in understanding family dynamics and psychological support, is essential for creating frameworks that not only accommodate an aging population but also uphold the principles of dignity, respect, and compassion. In this sense, effective end-of-life care systems can serve as a blueprint for addressing the implications of longevity beyond mere life extension. The intersection of cultural perspectives on death and dying further underscores the significance of end-of-life care in a future oriented toward increased longevity. Different societies hold diverse beliefs about death, influencing how they approach dying individuals and their families. Integrating these cultural perspectives into end-of-life care not only enriches the caregiving experience but also fosters a greater societal understanding of the complexities surrounding death. As aging populations become more diverse, health care practices need to adapt, ensuring that care providers are equipped to address the unique needs and values of various cultural groups. The images referenced in this analysis serve to illustrate the multifaceted aspects of end-of-life care, from the systemic changes required in healthcare practice to the importance of individualized approaches in light of diverse beliefs about aging and death. As we delve deeper into the uncharted territory of longevity, it becomes increasingly clear that a holistic approach to end-of-life care is not just a moral imperative but a necessity for maintaining the dignity and quality of life we aspire to extend through scientific innovation.

Year	Percentage of Adults with Advanced Care Plans	Percentage of Hospitals with Palliative Care Programs	Patient Satisfaction Score (1-10)
2020	46	72	8.5
2021	48	75	8.7
2022	50	78	8.9
2023	53	80	9

End-of-Life Care Quality Metrics

Advances in Pain Management

Emerging technologies and scientific advancements are revolutionizing the landscape of pain management, addressing a critical aspect that significantly impacts the quality of life as people age. One noteworthy area of development lies in the application of deep learning and artificial intelligence in personalizing pain treatment protocols. These innovations allow healthcare professionals to analyze vast datasets, including patient histories and genetic profiles, to tailor pain management strategies that are specifically suited to individual needs. By enabling more precise diagnoses and personalized interventions, such advancements not only enhance patient outcomes but also minimize reliance on opioids, mitigating the associated risks of dependency and adverse effects. This proactive approach emphasizes prevention and management strategies that accommodate the unique physiological and psychological aspects of each patient, aligning seamlessly with the broader goal of optimizing health as individuals extend their life spans. Such initiatives demonstrate a commitment to enhancing both physical and mental well-being in an aging population. Further developments in regenerative medicine offer significant promise for pain management through innovative therapies that address the underlying causes of pain rather than solely alleviating symptoms. Techniques such as stem cell therapy and platelet-rich plasma injections are emerging as viable treatments that encourage the repair and regeneration of damaged tissues. These therapies can rejuvenate joint function in osteoarthritis patients, providing pain relief while simultaneously restoring mobility and overall quality of life. Importantly, these advancements exemplify a shift from traditional pain management paradigms toward more holistic and sustainable solutions that promote healing at a cellular level. As regenerative approaches continue to evolve, they have the potential not only to improve physical health outcomes but also to contribute to the psychological well-being of patients experiencing chronic pain. This evolving landscape highlights the necessity of integrating such innovative treatments as vital components of a comprehensive strategy supporting longevity and an enhanced quality of life. The importance of interdisciplinary collaboration cannot be overstated in the context of advancing pain management techniques. By integrating knowledge from various fields, including neuroscience, pharmacology, and behavioral health, a more intricate understanding of pain mechanisms can be achieved. This collaborative approach facilitates the development of innovations such as digital health applications that enable real-time monitoring and management of pain conditions. Wearable technologies equipped with sensors can track biometrics, providing healthcare providers with crucial data to inform treatment adjustments. Such innovations align with the exploratory aims of maximizing human longevity by not only managing pain more effectively but also empowering patients to take an active role in their health journeys. As these efforts unfold, they pave the way for a comprehensive pain management paradigm that integrates technology, personal agency, and holistic treatment philosophies, exemplifying a critical shift toward fostering well-being amid the prospect of extended lifespans. References to images like and, which depict the interconnections between biological mechanisms and advances in health analysis, could significantly enhance the discussion of pain management technologies. They illustrate the underlying principles of personalizing treatments and regenerative therapies contributing to a more profound understanding of health, thus supporting the main argument of the essay. Incorporating imagery such as, which features advanced technology in healthcare, emphasizes the importance of digital health applications in pain management. By visualizing these critical advancements, the analysis can reinforce the overarching theme of the transformative nature of modern medicine as it aligns with the goal of living longer, healthier lives.

Holistic Approaches to Palliative Care

In the face of increasing life expectancy, the necessity for holistic approaches in palliative care becomes increasingly apparent. This model prioritizes comprehensive well-being by addressing not only the physical symptoms of terminal illnesses but also the emotional, spiritual, and social dimensions that significantly affect patients and their families. Traditional medical frameworks often emphasize disease eradication, which can inadvertently overlook the nuanced experiences of individuals nearing the end of life. By implementing a holistic approach, practitioners can create a support system that acknowledges patients as whole persons rather than just patients with diseases. This perspective fosters deeper connections between caregivers and patients, ultimately enhancing the quality of life through tailored management of pain and distress. Such integrative strategies will be essential as advancements in longevity medicine push the boundaries of life expectancy, ensuring that the extended years can be filled with dignity and fulfillment rather than mere survival. A holistic approach to palliative care encompasses a multidisciplinary team of professionals, which may include physicians, nurses, social workers, chaplains, and psychologists. Each team member brings a unique set of skills to address the diverse needs of patients. This collective effort ensures that all aspects of a patient's experience are considered, allowing for interventions that are not only symptomatically effective but also emotionally and socially supportive. The incorporation of patient and family preferences into care plans can also empower individuals, giving them a sense of control during an otherwise challenging time. Research indicates that holistic palliative care can lead to improved patient satisfaction, reduced anxiety, and even prolonged survival in some cases. As societal perspectives shift toward embracing the complexities of aging and end-of-life care, it becomes imperative that healthcare systems integrate these comprehensive methodologies to better serve their populations while acknowledging the individuality of each patient's journey. Cultural sensitivity plays a pivotal role in the effectiveness of holistic palliative care. Diverse beliefs and practices surrounding death and dying can significantly influence how patients and families experience the end of life. By recognizing and respecting these variances, healthcare providers can offer more empathetic and appropriate care. This inclusivity not only improves patient outcomes but also fosters trust between caregivers and families, thereby enhancing the therapeutic alliance. With the potential for extended life due to advancements in health and medicine, it is critical that palliative care evolves to accommodate these diverse cultural contexts, ensuring holistic approaches remain relevant and effective. The ongoing dialogue around these changes will shape future practices in palliative care, ultimately leading to a more compassionate, understanding, and responsive healthcare system as humanity grapples with the challenges of living longer lives. This conversation complements the increasing focus on quality of life, bringing to light the necessity of maintaining human dignity amidst potentially lengthy journeys through illness. In relation to the images referenced, images and would significantly enhance the analysis of Holistic Approaches to Palliative Care by illustrating the interconnectedness of biological aging, patient emotions, and systems biology, which are critical components in understanding the complexities of palliative care. These visuals will provide important context for discussing how holistic strategies can effectively integrate into practices designed for individuals undergoing care in the extended longevity landscape.

XXII. THE IMPACT OF LONGEVITY ON EDUCATION

Advancements in longevity have significant implications for the educational landscape, as the extended lifespan necessitates a re-evaluation of learning frameworks and curricula to accommodate lifelong learning. With individuals potentially living to 150 years, educational institutions may need to adopt more flexible models that allow for continuous skill acquisition and adaptation throughout a person's life. This implies a shift from traditional educational paradigms, which often confine learning to early life stages, toward a more dynamic and integrative approach. As depicted in, the interdisciplinary nature of modern biomedical research reflects a similar need in education; just as scientific fields integrate various domains, educational systems may benefit from weaving together diverse subjects to foster holistic understanding and adaptability. As the nature of work evolves due to technological advancements, preparing learners for multiple careers across their lifetimes will be imperative, necessitating an emphasis on critical thinking and adaptability in educational curricula. The societal implications of increased longevity will likely challenge educators to address varied learning needs across diverse age groups. As the workforce ages and older individuals seek to retrain or develop new skills, the role of educational institutions will expand beyond traditional age demographics, encompassing learners of all ages. This shift necessitates the development of educational environments that celebrate diversity in experience and knowledge, fostering mentorship opportunities where younger and older generations can share insights and skills. The interconnectedness of biological age and educational approaches, illustrated in, emphasizes the potential for cross-generational learning, where the life experiences of older adults inform and enrich the educational journey of younger individuals. By fostering these interactions, educational institutions can prepare society to thrive in a future where longevity not only extends life but also transforms the nature and purpose of education itself. The economic implications of longevity also underscore the need for an adaptive educational framework that emphasizes financial literacy and career readiness. As society faces an aging population that may require extended financial planning for retirement and healthcare, education systems must incorporate courses and programs focused on financial management, investment strategies, and healthy aging practices. The findings illustrated in regarding dietary influences on aging could also support educational programs that address health and wellness alongside financial planning, integrating holistic health into the curriculum. Preparing individuals to navigate the complexities of living longer lives means equipping them with tools to make informed decisions about their health and finances. Such an approach will not only enhance an individual's quality of life but also contribute to the economic resilience of communities, underscoring the vital role of education in creating a sustainable future in the face of increasing longevity.

Lifelong Learning Opportunities

As humanity aims to navigate the challenges of living significantly longer lives, the role of lifelong learning is increasingly pivotal. Embracing a continuous learning mindset can help individuals adapt to the rapid changes in technology and society that accompany increased longevity. Educational systems must evolve to offer accessible resources that cater to diverse age groups, enabling older adults to engage in skill development and knowledge acquisition. Such opportunities extend beyond conventional academic settings and include online platforms, community workshops, and intergenerational mentorship programs. By equipping people with the knowledge and skills necessary for adaptation, lifelong learning can empower individuals to thrive in an ever-evolving landscape, ultimately enhancing their quality of life as they age. Images like effectively illustrate the intersection of deep learning methodologies and health analysis, reinforcing the argument of how continuous education can unleash innovative approaches to healthcare and personal growth. Incorporating lifelong learning into the framework of aging requires an acknowledgment of the unique health challenges faced by older populations. Educational initiatives that focus on mental health, cognitive resilience, and physical wellbeing can foster healthier lifestyles and promote self-efficacy among seniors. Understanding the science of nutrition, exercise, and stress management can significantly affect biological aging and quality of life. Programs that offer training in utilizing technology can empower older adults to remain connected and informed, combating the isolation often associated with aging. Platforms such as virtual learning environments can facilitate knowledge sharing across generations, thus reinforcing community bonds. The representation provided in offers compelling insights into how childhood development impact biological aging, supporting the need for educational curricula that address health across a lifespan, effectively making lifelong learning a crucial ally in the quest for longevity. To prepare societies for a future where extended lifespans are the norm, it is necessary to cultivate a culture that values and promotes lifelong learning. This cultural shift relies heavily on recognizing the transformative potential learning possesses at all stages of life. Employers, educators, and community leaders must collaborate to create learning environments that cater to the varying needs of an aging populace, promoting personal development and employment opportunities well into later years. The integration of technology in learning facilitates greater access to resources and fosters innovative educational approaches that can be tailored to individual preferences and capabilities. To epitomize this fusion of education and modernization, serves as an effective depiction of systems-based approaches in biology and ecology, seamlessly connecting healthy practices to longevity. By embracing such collaborative and inclusive educational paradigms, society can not only prepare individuals for longer life but enrich their experience throughout the aging process.

Year	Adults Engaged in Learning (%)	Country
2020	36	United States
2021	40	Germany
2022	45	Japan
2023	38	United States
2023	50	Sweden
2023	42	Canada

Lifelong Learning Opportunities and Longevity

Educational Programs for Older Adults

As the aging population continues to grow, there is an increasing recognition of the need for educational programs tailored specifically for older adults. These initiatives not only provide opportunities for continued learning but also cultivate social engagement, which is vital for mental health and overall well-being. Research suggests that educational programs can enhance cognitive function and improve life satisfaction among older individuals. A range of activities, from digital literacy training to discussions about health and wellness, fosters a sense of community and belonging. By bridging generational gaps and facilitating knowledge exchange, these programs empower seniors to remain active participants in society, challenging age-related stereotypes that often diminish their capabilities. Emphasizing the importance of lifelong learning, such programs contribute to a culture that values the experience and wisdom of older adults, encouraging a more inclusive perspective on aging in contemporary society. serves as a compelling representation of this integration, showcasing how interdisciplinary approaches can enhance the learning landscape for seniors. Educational programs designed for older adults often embrace technology as a crucial component of the modern learning environment. Given the rapid pace of technological advancement, particularly in fields such as biotechnology and artificial intelligence, it is essential for older learners to acquire these skills. Interactive workshops and online courses can demystify technology, empowering seniors to navigate tools and platforms that increasingly pervade daily life. Such proficiency not only enhances their engagement with the world but also allows them to leverage technology for improved health management and social connectivity. Studies indicate that technological literacy in older adults positively correlates with better health outcomes, as seniors who are tech-savvy can access health information, connect with peers, and even participate in telemedicine. This points to a transformative potential that educational programs hold, enabling seniors to adapt to a hypothetical future in which technology plays an increasingly vital role in their lives. The interconnectedness of these learning experiences is echoed in, highlighting the role of continuous education in fostering adaptability among older adults. The effectiveness of educational programs for seniors also hinges on the incorporation of themes pertinent to their unique life experiences. Courses that delve into health and wellness, financial literacy, and even creative expression can resonate deeply with older adults, addressing their immediate concerns while inspiring personal growth. By focusing on relevant subject matter, these programs can enhance self-efficacy, equipping seniors with skills that enhance their independence and quality of life. Additionally, programs that encourage critical thinking and dialogue about aging can deepen participants understanding of their realities, ultimately cultivating resilience. This holistic approach ensures that educational initiatives remain meaningful and impactful, not merely serving as a means to pass time, but as vital tools for empowerment. Visualizing this multifaceted reality, illustrates how various lifestyle and educational frameworks collectively contribute to successful aging—a crucial consideration as society contemplates the implications of extending life expectancy for future generations.

Program Name	Participants (Annual)	Establishment Year	Country
University of the Third Age	200,000	1972	Global
Senior Learning Network	10,000	2003	United States
The Osher Lifelong Learning Institute	150,000	2001	United States
Road Scholar	150,000	1975	Global
Elderhostel	50,000	1995	Global

Educational Programs for Older Adults

Intergenerational Learning

In an era where life expectancy is expected to reach unprecedented lengths, the dynamic of knowledge transfer between generations becomes increasingly significant. Intergenerational learning promotes the sharing of knowledge, skills, and life experiences, facilitating a reciprocal relationship between younger and older individuals. As advancements in health and longevity reshape societal structures, the value of wisdom accumulated over decades cannot be understated. This knowledge becomes an invaluable resource for younger generations, enabling them to navigate complexities in a rapidly evolving world. Incorporating intergenerational learning into educational frameworks can bolster resilience and adaptability, equipping individuals to face future challenges with a broader understanding of historical and cultural contexts. This shared learning experience directly influences personal growth and development, creating a society that values contributions from all ages. Emphasizing these connections fosters a sense of community and belonging—crucial components for thriving in an extended lifespan. Such collaborations can also enhance the effectiveness of scientific and technological advancements, particularly in fields like regenerative medicine and biotechnology. The insights garnered from the lived experiences of older adults can guide researchers in developing age-related therapies that resonate with the needs of an aging population. Engaging in dialogues that respect and incorporate perspectives from diverse age groups can elevate the quality of scientific inquiry and inform better policy-making. This interactivity is especially relevant in the context of ethical considerations surrounding longevity; diverse viewpoints can yield more comprehensive and socially responsible solutions. By illustrating the importance of cross-generational involvement, communities can bolster public trust in innovations aimed at improving health outcomes. The diagram in captures the essence of this intergenerational synergy, presenting a framework that encompasses both the biological and psychological factors influencing health, thereby aligning health innovations with lessons from past experiences. Critically, intergenerational learning also plays a role in addressing societal concerns related to sustainability and quality of life as populations age. The collective wisdom of older generations can inform sustainable practices and adaptations that are essential for future living environments. Involving younger individuals in these discussions not only empowers them with historical knowledge but also inspires them to innovate responsibly, ensuring a balance between progress and ecological stewardship. As societies grapple with the implications of extended lifespans, intergenerational dialogue paves the way for cohesive action. By nurturing relationships across age groups, we can cultivate environments that support healthy aging while also addressing social disparities amplified by longer life expectancies. This concept is visualized in, which underscores the complexity of health determinants and the shared responsibility among different age cohorts in fostering sustainable development that benefits all.

XXIII. FUTURE RESEARCH DIRECTIONS IN LONGEVITY

Advancements in biotechnology and artificial intelligence are yielding unprecedented insights into the mechanisms of aging and longevity. Promising research avenues include the exploration of biological age markers, such as Methylation Profile Scores (MPSs), which may provide a deeper understanding of the aging process itself. Future studies could focus on refining these biomarkers to ascertain their predictive value for age-related diseases and overall health in various demographics. The integration of multi-omic approaches—encompassing genomics, proteomics, and metabolomics—could significantly enhance this research, enabling a comprehensive analysis of aging at both the molecular and systemic levels. As detailed in, these methodological innovations hold the potential to bridge the gap between early development and aging, helping researchers to identify crucial factors that impact health across the lifespan. By unraveling these complex interactions, scientists may unlock new strategies for promoting healthier aging and extending longevity. The ethical implications surrounding longevity research cannot be overlooked as these advancements progress. As society faces the feasibility of extending human life significantly, crucial questions arise about the ramifications for social structures, healthcare systems, and resource allocation. Public discourse must address whether societies are equipped to accommodate an aging population that could live well beyond the traditional life expectancy. Research initiatives should examine how longevity might impact intergenerational relationships, career trajectories, and economic stability within communities. As illustrated by the complexities depicted in, solutions should prioritize integration and equity, ensuring that advancements benefit diverse populations rather than exacerbating existing disparities. Addressing ethical considerations in parallel with technological innovations will be essential for guiding future research directions in longevity and fostering responsible advancements in health. An additional area of exploration lies in the socio-economic impacts of extended lifespans on sustainability and quality of life. Understanding how longer life expectancies might affect societal values, particularly regarding health, family dynamics, and individual purpose, is paramount. Research should delve into how changes in longevity influence lifestyle choices, such as diet and exercise, ultimately determining the quality of life as individuals age. The implications of these factors intersect with environmental sustainability, as longer life can increase the consumption of resources and generate further challenges in a world already grappling with issues such as climate change. As indicated by the insights from, interdisciplinary research that encompasses environmental science alongside gerontology will be crucial in developing sustainable practices that enhance longevity. By addressing these multifaceted issues holistically, future research can inform policies that promote not just longer life, but healthier and more fulfilling lives for all individuals, thus setting the stage for a more equitable and sustainable future.

Year	Source	Funding Amount
2019	National Institutes of Health (NIH)	$250 million
2020	National Institutes of Health (NIH)	$275 million
2021	National Institutes of Health (NIH)	300 million
2022	National Institutes of Health (NIH)	350 million
2023	National Institutes of Health (NIH)	400 million

Longevity Research Funding Trends

Emerging Fields of Study

The exploration of emerging fields like deep generative reinforcement learning is critical for understanding how advanced technologies can influence health outcomes and longevity. In recent years, this innovative approach has demonstrated remarkable potential in various biomedical applications, including precision medicine and molecular design. By harnessing the capabilities of artificial intelligence, researchers can analyze vast datasets, identifying patterns that contribute to our understanding of biological age and health throughout the lifecycle. Such techniques are not merely theoretical; they are being integrated into practical health applications, demonstrating that technologies once considered cutting-edge are rapidly becoming essential components of everyday medical practice. The schematic illustrated in aptly reflects how this convergence of biological research and computational analysis can lead to starker insights into health management, supporting the notion that a multidisciplinary approach is vital for navigating the complexities of longevity. Another pivotal area of exploration is the interface between nutrition and aging, particularly through dietary frameworks that directly influence health span and lifespan. Research has increasingly emphasized the significance of various dietary patterns—such as the ketogenic and Mediterranean diets—on cognitive function, inflammation, and overall wellness in older adults. These frameworks are not simply about the food we consume; they encompass a broader understanding of how lifestyle choices can mitigate age-related decline and enhance the quality of life. The findings represented in highlight the direct impacts of these diets on systemic health, framing nutrition as a powerful tool in the fight against the adverse effects of aging.

As such, the knowledge gleaned from nutritional studies is vital for developing comprehensive strategies that not only extend life expectancy but also improve the holistic health outcomes for individuals as they age. The integration of multi-omics analyses into aging research presents an exciting frontier in our understanding of longevity. By synthesizing data from genomics, proteomics, and metabolomics, scientists can construct intricate models that depict biological aging processes in real time. This cutting-edge field offers the potential to develop predictive biomarkers and personalized interventions, ultimately paving the way for targeted therapies that address the unique aging trajectories of individuals. The insights depicted through the image showcase how a multi-omic approach can synergize various biological layers to paint a detailed picture of aging mechanics. Such research underscores the complexity of human biology and positions these emerging technologies at the forefront of modern biomedical research, essential to fulfilling the promise of extended longevity while grappling with the associated ethical and societal challenges.

Field	Current Impact	Projected Growth
Genetics	Understanding genetic factors that influence aging processes	Increased advancement in gene therapies and CRISPR technology
Regenerative Medicine	Innovative treatments such as stem cell therapy and tissue engineering	Potential for growing organs and tissues for transplantation
Artificial Intelligence in Healthcare	AI applications improving diagnostics and patient care	Expansion of AI tools to predict health outcomes and personalize treatment
Nutrigenomics	Study of how diet affects gene expression and aging	Emerging personalized nutrition plans to prolong healthy lifespan
Microbiome Research	Understanding the relationship between gut health and aging	Potential insights into preventive strategies for age-related diseases

Emerging Fields of Study in Longevity Research

Interdisciplinary Approaches

Integrating multiple disciplines is not merely an academic exercise; it is a necessity for comprehensively addressing the challenges associated with increased longevity. The intersection of fields such as biology, data science, and psychology reveals intricate relationships that are pivotal to the understanding of aging and health. Advancements in deep generative reinforcement learning, as illustrated in image, demonstrate how complex data from genomics and proteomics can be harnessed to refine predictive models for biological age and health status. This interdisciplinary approach allows researchers to tap into vast datasets, deriving insights that are unattainable through traditional methodologies. The consolidation of various scientific domains leads to innovative solutions in precision medicine, ultimately aiming to enhance individual health outcomes and extend healthy life years, thus representing a transformative step toward achieving the goal of living longer, healthier lives. The examination of childhood development in relation to aging underscores the importance of an interdisciplinary framework that encompasses developmental biology and psychological health. Image presents a conceptual model that elucidates the connection between methylation profile scores (MPSs) and both biological aging processes and early life development. By understanding how childhood experiences influence aging, researchers can better formulate interventions aimed at promoting lifelong health. This integrated approach signifies a paradigm shift in how we view health; rather than treating aging as a linear trajectory, it perceives it as a complex interplay of early developmental factors that may predispose individuals to age-related conditions. Such insights validate the necessity of collaborative research that blends disciplines such as genetics, environmental science, and mental health to develop comprehensive health strategies for future generations. As the prospect of extending human life significantly challenges existing societal norms, the role of interdisciplinary research becomes increasingly vital in informing policy and ethical considerations. The analysis depicted in image highlights various dietary approaches and their effects on aging, demonstrating that solutions to longevity will not be found in isolation. The myriad factors influencing longevity—ranging from nutrition and cognitive function to social interactions—call for cohesive strategies that embrace insights from diverse fields, including sociology, nutrition science, and psychology. Addressing the complexities of life extension demands a collective understanding of how individual choices resonate within broader societal frameworks. Interdisciplinary collaboration, therefore, not only enhances scientific inquiry but also prepares society for the implications of extended lifespans, fostering a culture that is equipped to navigate the challenges and opportunities that accompany longer life expectancy.

Funding and Support for Research

The allocation of funding and support for research is crucial in advancing the frontiers of human longevity. Diverse funding sources, encompassing federal grants, private investments, non-profit organizations, and international collaborations, drive the exploration of life-extending technologies. Specific initiatives funded by government entities, such as the National Institutes of Health (NIH), focus on regenerative medicine and aging biology, directly influencing the pace and scope of research in these areas. Philanthropic contributions, particularly from affluent individuals and foundations, play a significant role in supporting innovative projects that may not fit conventional funding criteria. These financial resources enable researchers to explore uncharted territories such as deep generative reinforcement learning in biomedical applications, as illustrated in. By analyzing how different funding mechanisms operate in synergy, it becomes evident that a collaborative framework is essential to accelerating the development of groundbreaking therapies that may one day facilitate living healthy lives well into our 150s. In addition to financial aspects, the infrastructure supporting research initiatives entails robust organizational and networking frameworks. Collaborations across academic institutions, industry players, and governmental agencies foster interdisciplinary approaches that enhance the efficacy of scientific inquiry. The emergence of global research consortia attests to the growing importance of shared knowledge and resources in tackling complex issues like aging. These alliances allow researchers to pool expertise and data, yielding comprehensive studies that drive the development of innovative healthcare solutions. The systems biology approach depicted in underscores the value of integrating multiple disciplines to better understand the multifaceted nature of aging and its related diseases. Such collaborative environments not only expedite discoveries but also broaden the impact of research outcomes, ensuring a greater societal benefit. Establishing a culture that promotes cooperation while effectively utilizing funds is vital for addressing the challenges posed by an aging population. Ethical considerations surrounding funding and support for research must be part of the broader discourse on longevity advancements. The potential for conflicts of interest in funding sources raises questions about the motivations that drive research agendas and outcomes. Transparency in funding processes and the prioritization of public health over profit are crucial for maintaining scientific integrity. Research funded by pharmaceutical companies may lean toward profitable interventions rather than equitable solutions that benefit broader populations, complicating the quest for effective aging therapies. The ethical frameworks illustrated in provide guidance on navigating these concerns and ensuring that advancements in science serve the public good. Addressing these ethical dilemmas will be increasingly vital as we venture toward a future where prolonging life becomes not just a possibility but a societal norm, ensuring that quality of life and health at extended ages are paramount in all research initiatives.

XXIV. CASE STUDIES OF LONGEVITY

Throughout history, significant demographic studies have revealed compelling insights into the factors contributing to longevity, with various populations exhibiting remarkable lifespans due to specific lifestyle choices, cultural practices, and environmental conditions. One notable case study includes the residents of the Blue Zones—regions marked by high concentrations of centenarians, such as Sardinia and Okinawa. Research indicates that these communities prioritize plant-based diets, regular physical activity, strong social connections, and a sense of purpose, which together foster not only longevity but also enhanced quality of life. The data underscore the intricacies of aging, suggesting that physical and mental well-being are closely intertwined and must be cultivated holistically. As we examine these cases, we can glean strategies to promote longevity that extend beyond mere biological interventions, indicating that societal frameworks and lifestyle adaptations play crucial roles in nurturing a sustainable approach to living longer, healthier lives. In addition to lifestyle and cultural dimensions, cutting-edge research in biotechnology and genetic editing is increasingly shaping our understanding of longevity by targeting the biological mechanisms of aging. Recent advancements in fields like regenerative medicine and gene therapy offer promising avenues for mitigating age-related decline. Stem cell therapies demonstrate potential in rejuvenating damaged tissues and organs, effectively reversing some of the biological changes associated with aging. The exploration of longevity genes—such as those found in model organisms like nematodes and mice—opens new discussions about the underlying genetic factors that regulate lifespan. Compelling case studies from organisms exhibiting exceptional longevity contribute to our knowledge of how similar principles may be applied in humans. As we advance our grasp of these scientific principles, the dialogue surrounding the ethical implications of such interventions is critical, as society must navigate questions of access, inequality, and the potential impacts of extending life on social structures and resources. The intersection of scientific research and cultural perceptions of aging further complicates the narrative around longevity. Different societies not only have varying attitudes towards aging but also diverse approaches to healthcare and wellness that influence life expectancy. While Western societies often regard aging as a decline, Mediterranean cultures emphasize respect for the elderly and their integration within family structures, which has been shown to correlate with improved health outcomes and longevity. Such case studies reveal the influences of social determinants of health that contribute to life expectancy and prompt essential discussions about the implications of longevity on politics, economics, and everyday life. As nations grapple with aging populations, the lessons learned from varying cultural contexts may guide policymakers in developing comprehensive strategies that embrace the holistic well-being of their citizens. A multidisciplinary approach that incorporates insights from longevity studies can help envision a future where living to 150 years becomes a realistic goal that enhances societal welfare and individual fulfillment.

Blue Zones and Their Secrets

Cultural practices play a crucial role in understanding the tenacity of Blue Zones, regions where people enjoy extraordinary longevity. These communities—such as those in Sardinia, Italy and Okinawa, Japan—share lifestyle elements that significantly contribute to their inhabitants' lifespan. Common threads include diets rich in plant-based foods, physical activity integrated into daily routines, and strong social connections that foster a sense of belonging. The Mediterranean diet emphasizes whole grains, legumes, and healthy fats, particularly olive oil, which are known to reduce inflammation and promote heart health. The importance of communal gatherings goes beyond nourishment; they create environments that encourage emotional support and mental well-being. The integration of these cultural norms offers a blueprint for changing modern lifestyles, suggesting that adopting similar practices could enhance longevity worldwide. Such observations underscore the potential for cultural adaptation in the pursuit of longer, healthier lives. This transformative lifestyle approach is captured eloquently in the insights from, which details the positive outcomes associated with deep learning methodologies that can analyze dietary patterns and social behaviors. The biological underpinnings of aging as manifested in Blue Zones are equally significant. Research indicates that genetic factors can enhance resilience against age-related diseases, but environmental and lifestyle choices predominantly dictate health outcomes. The centenarians in Ikaria, Greece, famously exhibit lower rates of dementia and chronic diseases, possibly due to their active lifestyles, mental engagement, and consumption of antioxidant-rich foods. Studies have identified critical biological mechanisms, including the role of omega-3 fatty acids from fish and the benefits of regular physical activity on cardiovascular health, which contribute to aging well. This multi-faceted approach to aging, combining genetics, environment, and lifestyle, emphasizes the need for a comprehensive understanding of longevity. The rich biology of these communities sheds light on the interconnectedness of various health factors, as depicted in, which illustrates the aging processes in a visual manner that underlines the significance of systematic biological interventions in health span extension. Building upon the cultural and biological dimensions of longevity, the socioeconomic contexts within Blue Zones provide additional layers of understanding. These regions often exhibit lower levels of stress and more equitable resource distributions, which contribute to enhanced mental and physical health. In Costa Rica's Nicoya Peninsula, people prioritize family, community, and active social engagement, which reduces loneliness and improves mental health—a significant factor in longevity. The socio-political environment promotes access to healthcare and social services, which enables healthier aging. Citizens in these areas often possess a strong sense of purpose, described as ikigai in Japanese culture, suggesting that having a reason to wake up every day plays a vital role in longevity. This perspective aligns with the broader narrative explored in, which juxtaposes individual and community health determinants, emphasizing the complex interplay of social factors in achieving a long and fulfilling life. Integrating these lessons could pave the way for innovative policies promoting health equity and lifestyle adjustments critical for increasing longevity on a larger scale.

Successful Aging Models

The concept of successful aging models encompasses a multifaceted approach, recognizing that aging is not merely the absence of disease but a complex interplay of various physical, psychological, and social factors. Successful aging models emphasize the importance of maintaining functional ability, cognitive health, and emotional well-being as pivotal indicators of life satisfaction in later years. Emerging research in fields such as gerontology and psychology has highlighted frameworks that prioritize adaptive strategies to navigate aging's challenges. The emphasis on resilience and the ability to engage in purposeful activities can significantly enhance quality of life during the aging process. Integrating these models into healthcare practices could lead to a paradigm shift where the focus transcends the traditional biomedical model, ultimately fostering environments conducive to healthy aging. The relevance of this paradigm is underscored by, which illustrates applications of deep generative reinforcement learning in health analysis, emphasizing how innovative data-driven approaches can inform strategies for successful aging. Complementing these models is the understanding that social determinants, such as socioeconomic status and community engagement, play a crucial role in successful aging. It is increasingly evident that accessing resources, social networks, and opportunities for meaningful participation directly impacts health outcomes for older adults. Successful aging is, therefore, not solely an individual endeavor; it necessitates collective societal efforts to create inclusive environments that support the aging population. Anticipating the challenges posed by an aging society, particularly in areas like healthcare accessibility and age-friendly community development, is vital in aligning national policies with the needs of older adults. This shift highlights the relationship between social support systems and individual aging experiences, which is poignantly reflected in. This image effectively summarizes the interconnected health determinants that influence successful aging, reinforcing the idea that a holistic approach is essential for fostering longevity. The implementation of technological advancements offers promising avenues for enhancing successful aging models. Innovations in biotechnology, such as telemedicine and wearable health technologies, empower older individuals to manage their health proactively and maintain connectivity with healthcare providers. These advancements not only facilitate more personalized care but also promote independence and autonomy, integral components of successful aging. The introduction of such technology also raises critical questions regarding equity and accessibility, as not all aging populations may have equal access to these advancements. Addressing disparities will be key to ensuring that technological progress benefits all segments of an aging population. By understanding and integrating these factors into successful aging models, society can better prepare for the complexities of longevity. This integrative perspective is further supported by, which outlines various dietary approaches impacting health outcomes and emphasizes the importance of a multi-faceted strategy involving nutrition, activity, and social engagement in enhancing the aging experience.

Model	Location	Life Expectancy (Years)	Key Factors
The Blue Zones	Various (Okinawa, Sardinia, etc.)	90+	Diet, social engagement, active lifestyle
Dan Buettner's 9 Lessons	Global	Varies	Purpose, stress reduction, plant-based diet
Aging Well Program	USA	80+	Health screenings, community support, physical activity
Swedish Model	Sweden	83	Social welfare programs, healthcare access, quality of life
Japan's Elderly Care	Japan	85	Family support, physical exercise, nutrition
Health at Every Size	USA	Varies	Body positivity, balanced nutrition, active lifestyles

Successful Aging Models Data

Lessons from Centenarians

Lessons derived from the lives of centenarians underscore essential lifestyle choices that contribute to longevity and well-being. These individuals often exhibit remarkable resilience and adaptability, revealing the significance of social connections and a sense of purpose. Many centenarians emphasize the importance of maintaining relationships with family and friends, showcasing the role of social interaction in promoting mental and emotional health. Research highlights that these social bonds can even mitigate stress and enhance quality of life, an insight vital in our understanding of aging. The interconnectedness of physical activity and mental engagement emerges as a common thread in their narratives, illustrating how an active lifestyle, whether through structured exercise or informal daily activities, is pivotal to functional longevity. Drawing from these observations can shape future frameworks for promoting health in an aging society and inform interventions aimed at improving health outcomes as more individuals reach advanced ages. A profound aspect of the centenarian experience lies in their relationship with food and nutrition, which frequently emphasizes moderation and balance. These long-lived individuals often follow diets rich in whole foods, including fruits, vegetables, and lean proteins, while limiting processed foods and added sugars. Portions are often smaller, and meals are consumed mindfully, reflecting cultural practices that prioritize community dining and slow eating. The Mediterranean diet, often common among centenarians in that region, highlights how dietary patterns can align with longevity principles and overall health outcomes. These shared dietary habits echo the sentiments of the observational studies linking diet quality with reduced risks of chronic diseases, underscoring the powerful role of nutrition in lifespan extension. Considering the implications of these dietary insights can guide future nutritional guidelines and public health strategies aimed at promoting healthier eating practices across age groups, particularly in the context of increasing life expectancy. To visualize the impact of nutrition on centenarian health, the insights observed in part (a) of serve as a clear example of how dietary practices are intricately tied to overall well-being. The mental fortitude exhibited by centenarians reveals critical lessons about resilience and positive mindset in the face of adversity. Many long-lived individuals attribute their longevity to a robust outlook on life and the ability to cope with stressors effectively. They often embrace change and view challenges as opportunities for growth, representing a profound psychological approach to aging. This adaptability not only fosters a lower incidence of mental health issues but also enables ongoing personal development and engagement in life's pursuits. Understanding the psychological dimensions of longevity provides essential context for designing interventions that nurture mental health, particularly as society braces for the implications of an aging population. The strategies gleaned from centenarian resilience contribute to a broader discourse on promoting mental wellness in older adults, aligning closely with the themes of sustained engagement and purpose explored within the essay. As evidenced by the life stories captured in, these psychological attributes are instrumental to both personal health and societal investment in longevity-focused initiatives.

Age	Country	Life Expectancy	Health Factors
100	Japan	84.6	Diet, exercise, community support
101	Italy	83.5	Mediterranean diet, family ties
102	United States	78.5	Access to healthcare, social engagement
103	Australia	82.5	Active lifestyle, clean environment
104	France	79.4	Balanced diet, mental stimulation
105	Canada	81.2	Regular physical activity, healthy weight

Centenarian Life Expectancy and Factors

XXV. PUBLIC PERCEPTION OF LONGEVITY

Public discussions surrounding longevity reveal a complex interplay between scientific advancements and societal values. As breakthroughs in biotechnology and genetic engineering suggest the potential for extended lifespans, varying opinions arise among different demographics. Older generations, for instance, may cherish the prospect of additional years filled with wisdom and experience, while younger individuals often express concerns regarding the implications of such longevity on their own opportunities and life trajectories. The perception of living significantly longer than the current average life expectancy is shaped not just by scientific potential but also by cultural, ethical, and financial considerations. These factors shape how individuals and communities envision their future, pointing to a need for deeper dialogues about what extended life truly means. Challenges related to the quality of life in prolonged lifespans significantly influence perceptions of longevity. While extended life expectancy presents enticing possibilities, questions about health quality, mental well-being, and societal roles in later years complicate the narrative. The fear of living longer in an increasingly dependent state resonates strongly, especially in societies that struggle with age-related health issues. People often wonder, What is the value of living to 150 if it means prolonged suffering or loss of autonomy? This outlook is compounded by the current state of healthcare systems and the availability of supportive resources for aging populations. The perceived efficacy of medical innovations can directly impact public sentiment, emphasizing the importance of creating a robust infrastructure that can accommodate both health and societal needs as lifespans extend. The interrelation between health outcomes and public perception of longevity must be addressed holistically. The evolving landscape of societal dynamics in response to longevity also merits scrutiny. As the potential for extended lifespans becomes more tangible, discussions warrant exploration of how family structures, work environments, and community engagements may transform. In cultures that place significant importance on youth, longer life could shift intergenerational relationships, potentially leading to conflict over resources and opportunities. Conversely, in some cultures, longer life might be embraced, leading to a greater reverence for elder wisdom and experience. Additionally, industries might be compelled to innovate in creating environments that support multigenerational interaction. As evidenced by the connections in various research domains, the future of longevity is a multifaceted issue deserving of careful discourse that reflects diverse cultural views and practical implications. Images such as and serve as conduits for understanding these dynamics, visually encapsulating how deep generative reinforcement learning intersects with aging and public health perceptions, underpinning the potential impact on longevity.

Media Representation of Aging

Media representation plays a crucial role in shaping societal perceptions of aging, oftentimes reflecting deep-seated stereotypes and cultural narratives. The portrayal of older adults in various forms of media can perpetuate ageism, presenting aging individuals as frail, dependent, or out of touch with contemporary culture. This reductive viewpoint fails to acknowledge the complexity and diversity of the aging population, who may possess vitality, wisdom, and an eagerness to engage with new technologies and ideas. Effective media representation should move beyond these simplistic archetypes, instead focusing on the nuanced experiences of individuals who defy these stereotypes. An example is reflected in, where the integration of advanced technology in healthcare settings points to a shift in how aging is represented, emphasizing collaboration between the younger and older working cohorts and framing aging within a context of capability and potential rather than decline. The advancements in biotechnology and regenerative medicine hold the potential to revolutionize the aging experience, yet media portrayals often lag behind the realities of these innovations. This disconnection creates an obstacle for public understanding and acceptance of longer life spans and enhanced health in older age. Cinematic and literary narratives frequently depict aging as synonymous with deterioration rather than evolution, which can evoke fear or resistance to embracing a future where life expectancy may extend significantly. A critical examination of these narratives highlights the need for stories that celebrate the possibilities of aging, such as those illustrated in, where interdisciplinary approaches to precision medicine demonstrate how science can empower individuals to live healthier lives as they age. By depicting these advancements positively, media can help catalyze a cultural shift in attitudes toward aging, promoting a more optimistic outlook on longevity. Cultural attitudes towards aging vary significantly across societies, and media representations can either amplify or challenge these perspectives. In some cultures, the elderly are revered for their knowledge and experience, while in others, they may be marginalized. Understanding these variances is essential for creating media that respects cultural differences while promoting a global conversation about aging and longevity. Comparative analyses of media representations are instrumental in uncovering how these nuances manifest across various platforms. Using images such as, which explores dietary approaches related to aging, provides insight into how lifestyle factors are depicted within different cultural contexts and their impact on the perception of the aging process. Such representations can help to deconstruct stereotypes and encourage a more inclusive dialogue that recognizes the rich tapestry of experiences associated with aging, ultimately fostering a society better prepared to address the challenges of living longer lives.

Public Awareness Campaigns

In an era where advances in biotechnology and medical research are poised to redefine human boundaries, public awareness campaigns play a crucial role in shaping societal perspectives on longevity. Such campaigns serve not only as platforms for disseminating scientific knowledge but also as means to engage the public in dialogue about the implications of extended life expectancy. While emerging technologies, such as genetic editing and regenerative medicine, promise transformative benefits, they also raise critical ethical concerns. By fostering understanding and stimulating discussions, public awareness initiatives can help mitigate fears and foster a sense of preparedness among citizens. Campaigns can address misconceptions about aging and the related technologies, ensuring that discussions remain grounded in evidence-based information. The visual representation of these interactions, as seen in, underscores the interconnectedness of deep generative reinforcement learning applications in biomedical research, showcasing the potential benefits and responsibilities that come with increased longevity. Effective public awareness campaigns have the potential to bridge the gap between scientific advancements and societal readiness for impending changes in longevity. By educating diverse demographics about the nuances of health promotion and disease prevention, these initiatives can empower individuals to take an active role in shaping their futures. Campaigns can draw on a variety of communication strategies, from traditional media to social media platforms, to reach a broader audience and stimulate engagement. A focused approach that emphasizes positive health behaviors, as illustrated in, demonstrates the interconnected nature of biological factors and lifestyle choices, providing practical guidance while underscoring the relevance of individual decision-making in contributing to broader health outcomes. Integrating insights from various fields can help ensure that the narrative surrounding longer life spans is constructive and accessible, ultimately positioning the public as informed stakeholders in discussions concerning life extension technologies. The cultural context greatly influences the effectiveness of public awareness campaigns tailored to longevity. Different cultures may have unique perspectives on aging, health, and quality of life, which can shape public receptivity to new ideas surrounding extended lifespan. Through culturally sensitive approaches, campaigns can address distinct values and norms, thereby enhancing their impact within specific communities. By emphasizing the role of community and familial support systems in navigating the complexities of longer life, such campaigns can cultivate a more inclusive dialogue. The frameworks presented in highlight the importance of transdisciplinary research, wherein insights from psychology and biology converge to inform public discourse. Recognizing the diverse narratives that surround aging will enable societal engagement on this topic, helping to build resilience and adaptability as humanity faces the potential reality of living well beyond traditional expectations of lifespan.

Year	Campaign Name	Target Audience	Awareness Level Percentage	Key Message
2021	Longevity Matters	Adults 30-50	45	Importance of healthy lifestyles for longevity
2022	Live Longer, Live Well	Seniors 60+	60	Benefits of regular health check-ups
2023	Future of Longevity	General Public	55	Understanding advancements in health and technology

Public Awareness Campaigns Awareness Statistics

Attitudes Toward Longevity Technologies

The intersection of scientific innovation and public perception significantly shapes the landscape of longevity technologies. As advancements in biotechnology, regenerative medicine, and genetic editing progress, the publics attitudes toward these technologies vary widely. Some embrace the potential for extended lifespans, viewing age extension as a pathway to further personal achievements and life experiences. This perspective aligns with the optimistic narrative surrounding new developments, such as those portrayed in, which showcases innovations in precision medicine and molecular design. Conversely, others voice skepticism or ethical concerns, questioning the desirability and implications of drastically extending human life. The fear of exacerbating existing inequalities, and the potential depletion of resources, reflect a collective wariness that must be addressed. Thus, understanding these diverse attitudes is essential for stakeholders in the field to foster informed discussions and create technologies harmonized with societal values. In considering the societal implications of longevity technologies, the focus must extend beyond individual perspectives to how communities and cultures interpret the prospect of extended lifespan. Various societal constructs influence acceptance or resistance to these advancements. Cultures that prioritize youth and vitality might view longevity technologies favorably, perceiving them as enhancements to an already vibrant existence. In contrast, societies that revere wisdom and experience may approach these innovations with caution, viewing them through the lens of historical context and moral implications. Insights gleaned from the cellular mechanisms of aging, such as those depicted in, can educate the public about the biological processes involved in aging, potentially shifting discussions toward a more informed, nuanced understanding. By promoting an interdisciplinary dialogue that incorporates cultural values, stakeholders can better navigate the complexities of societal attitudes toward longevity, ultimately allowing innovations to resonate more fully with the broader public. The economic implications of longevity technologies intertwine significantly with public sentiment and societal readiness for these advancements. As the prospect of longer lives becomes tangible through cutting-edge science, questions about the sustainability of healthcare systems, workforce dynamics, and resource allocation arise. The integration of longevity technologies into everyday life could lead to enhanced productivity and economic growth, as indicated in, showcasing the potential positive outcomes for society. The economic burden of an aging population, characterized by increased healthcare costs and pension pressures, cannot be ignored. Public perception thus plays a pivotal role; if society is receptive to these technologies and the changes they bring, it may lead to favorable policy frameworks and resource allocations. Conversely, if skepticism prevails, this could hinder innovation and exacerbate economic inequalities across various demographics. Addressing these economic concerns through transparent communication and community engagement is vital to building a society that is genuinely prepared for the ramifications of living significantly longer lives.

Age Group	Support Percentage	Concern Percentage	Neutral Percentage
18-24	62	15	23
25-34	70	12	18
35-44	60	20	20
45-54	55	25	20
55-64	50	30	20
65+	45	35	20

Attitudes Toward Longevity Technologies

XXVI. CONCLUSION

In contemplating the potential for extending human life to 150 years, it is crucial to synthesize the myriad factors influencing this ambitious prospect. The advancements in deep generative reinforcement learning, as denoted in, are beginning to shape our understanding of health and aging. They offer a glimpse into how intelligent algorithms can improve precision medicine and personalize treatments based on individual health trajectories. Such technologies not only provide a foundation for effective medical interventions but also raise questions about the scalability of these practices across different demographic groups. As society considers the ramifications of aging populations, the integration of these sophisticated methodologies may play a pivotal role in ensuring that longevity translates to enhanced quality of life rather than merely extending the years lived. The convergence of technology and biology, therefore, becomes essential in redefining health standards and practices for a society grappling with an unprecedented life expectancy. As we analyze our readiness for such longevity, it becomes evident that cultural and ethical considerations must accompany scientific advancements. Social frameworks and perceptions of aging vary widely across cultures, as portrayed in. The concept of an aging clock, which recognizes different biological and chronological aging processes, presents a challenge to conventional views of gerontology. It emphasizes the need for a culturally nuanced understanding of longevity, as societies may have differing values regarding health, vitality, and societal contributions in their later years. The ethical dilemmas posed by extending life, from resource allocation to quality of care, require deep collective reflection. Thus, addressing these challenges not only involves medical and technological readiness but also necessitates an ongoing dialogue about how society values the lives of its older members and how it can adapt to their evolving roles. Considering the economic implications of a 150-year lifespan, the dynamics of work and family structures are poised for a fundamental shift. The integration of multi-omics approaches in aging research, as indicated in, reveals the complex interplay between biological aging and socio-economic factors. This interplay is critical in predicting the future workforce, where longer life could mean longer careers but also necessitate new forms of retirement and social support systems. Additionally, as families navigate longer generational overlaps, traditional roles may evolve, impacting caregiving, and familial support. Preparing society for longevity entails not only embracing scientific and technological advancements but also rethinking economic models and social safety nets that accommodate an aging populace. Through robust discourse and strategic planning, society can better equip itself for the consequences of prolonged life, ensuring that extended years are filled with purpose, health, and fulfillment.

Summary of Key Findings

Recent advancements in biotechnology and genomics pave the way for innovative approaches to understanding aging and longevity. Research into methylation profile scores (MPSs) has illuminated the connection between epigenetic changes and biological aging processes, revealing potential pathways to mitigate age-related decline. The prospective development of new MPSs tailored to childhood development reflects a growing recognition of the interplay between early life experiences and lifelong health. Collectively, these findings underscore the significance of early interventions and the need to revisit our understanding of aging, suggesting that proactive strategies could significantly enhance the quality of life for individuals as they age. The implications of these insights encourage a reevaluation of how society approaches both preventive health measures and opportunities for extending life, which can be particularly crucial as the quest for longevity evolves. These complex relationships warrant significant attention in ongoing discussions of health optimization as society navigates the possibilities of extended lifespans. Exploring dietary influences highlights how lifestyle choices can affect biological aging, emphasizing the need for holistic approaches to health. Evidence suggests that dietary patterns, including the ketogenic and Mediterranean diets, contribute positively to health outcomes such as weight management and cognitive function. These findings correlate with observed reductions in biological aging markers, linking nutrition with longevity and overall well-being. As society becomes increasingly aware of the significance of diet in health maintenance, these insights will shape the conversation around preventive health strategies. Additionally, integrating dietary sciences within the broader frame of health research can foster effective public health policies aimed at longevity. The acknowledgment of dietary factors offers a tangible avenue for individuals and communities striving for healthier living and longevity, reinforcing the interconnectedness of lifestyle choices and aging. Encouraging healthy dietary habits can thus play a pivotal role in the larger narrative concerning human longevity, presenting actionable solutions for enhancing individual health as life expectancy increases. Technological innovations in deep generative reinforcement learning and systems biology represent a transformative shift in how aging research is conducted. These advancements empower scientists to model complex biological interactions and predict outcomes more accurately, enhancing our understanding of aging mechanisms. The interdisciplinary nature of this research, as highlighted by various projects, underscores the growing recognition that aging is not merely an individual process but rather a multifaceted phenomenon influenced by genetic, environmental, and socio-economic factors. The integration of systems biology with machine learning techniques propels research forward, enabling more effective design and implementation of interventions aimed at promoting longevity. Such innovations could potentially redefine societal structures, influencing everything from healthcare systems to individual lifestyle choices. In light of these findings, the readiness to embrace a future of extended lifespans becomes increasingly plausible, yet necessitates a comprehensive approach to ensure that advancements in technology are matched with ethical considerations and equitable health access.

Implications for Society

As humanity inches closer to the prospect of prolonging life well beyond current limits, societal frameworks must adapt to accommodate shifting demographics and evolving health paradigms. With advancements in biotechnology and regenerative medicine heralding the possibility of significantly extended lifespans, society faces the challenge of integrating older populations into both social structures and the workforce. The significant variation in aging processes, as illustrated by the concept of aging clocks linking health metrics to biological age, complicates the narrative further. It suggests that a one-size-fits-all approach to aging will be impractical. As a result, societies may need to rethink how they structure retirement, healthcare, and employment policies to ensure that older individuals remain productive and engaged while being supported adequately. This necessitates comprehensive policy discussions to ensure economic implications are addressed, promoting intergenerational cooperation rather than competition for resources. Additionally, prolonging life alters the societal fabric and cultural perception of age. Traditionally, culture has dictated a sequence of life stages where youth is revered, and old age is often marginalized. Nonetheless, if extended longevity becomes a reality, this perception could shift significantly. The reconfiguration of family structures may also ensue, as elder family members might play more active roles in caregiving for younger generations, leading to a richer familial support dynamic. Consequently, communities may need to foster new norms that celebrate and leverage the wisdom and experience of older individuals, facilitating societal integration rather than isolation. Shifting societal values could reshape expectations regarding age-appropriate behavior and openness toward multi-generational living, fostering environments where age diversity is embraced. The ethical implications surrounding extended lifespans cannot be sidelined, as they raise pertinent questions about equity and access to life-extending technologies. The potential for disparities to arise, where only affluent individuals can afford advanced medical treatments prolonging life, poses a serious threat to social cohesion. This inequality may breed discontent and conflict, challenging the foundational principles of fairness and justice that societies strive to uphold. If the distribution of longevity technologies remains unequal, societal divisions could deepen, exacerbating existing challenges related to healthcare access and economic viability. Frameworks that promote equitable access must be developed alongside technological advancements to ensure that everyone, regardless of socioeconomic status, has the opportunity to benefit from increased longevity. Addressing these concerns requires proactive dialogue and inclusive policy-making to harmonize technological advancements with ethical principles that safeguard social justice.

Future Outlook on Longevity

The landscape of longevity is rapidly evolving, shaped by scientific breakthroughs and cultural shifts that promise a redefinition of human life expectancy. Groundbreaking research in fields such as biotechnology and regenerative medicine underscores the potential for extending life through innovative therapies. Techniques like genome editing and cellular rejuvenation are not merely theoretical; they are beginning to infiltrate clinical practices, suggesting that age-related diseases may one day become manageable or even preventable. Advancements in methylation profile scores (MPSs) can help evaluate biological age by analyzing DNA methylation patterns, as highlighted in. This framework could revolutionize how we perceive aging, moving from a focus solely on chronological age to a more nuanced understanding of biological health. Such developments offer not just the prospect of longer lives but also the potential for healthier lifespans, where individuals can thrive well into their 150s, fundamentally altering societal perspectives on aging. As we contemplate the implications of extended life, it is essential to recognize the accompanying ethical and social challenges that will inevitably arise. The prospect of living significantly longer encompasses not just individual health but also the broader societal context, including family structures, workforce dynamics, and economic implications. If life expectancy increases, traditional career pathways could be disrupted, necessitating a reevaluation of retirement age, savings, and healthcare resources. The integration of diverse cultures views on aging, as discussed in, highlights a patchwork of acceptance and resistance, shaping public policy and personal approaches to longevity. Discussions surrounding equity in health access and the potential for increased strain on social services must be explored to ensure that extending life leads to enhanced quality of life rather than exacerbated inequalities. The environmental sustainability of prolonged lifespans cannot be overlooked, as the challenges of managing larger populations become increasingly pronounced. Questions arise regarding resource allocation, environmental impact, and planetary health when a significant portion of society is living considerably longer. Investigating dietary interventions and lifestyle changes, as suggested by the relationships between dietary patterns and aging in, offers promising insights into promoting healthy longevity while minimizing ecological footprints. Societal adaptations need to align with sustainable practices that support not just the health of individuals but also the well-being of the planet. As we venture deeper into this age of longevity, interdisciplinary approaches encompassing ethics, economics, and environmental stewardship will be critical in ensuring that the pursuit of extended life becomes a holistic endeavor, benefitting both humanity and the Earth.

Final Thoughts on Readiness for Extended Life

The prospect of living significantly longer lives presents both remarkable potential and considerable challenges. As we advance in biotechnology, regenerative medicine, and genetic editing, the scientific landscape is evolving rapidly. Achieving longevity requires more than just technological breakthroughs; social and ethical implications loom as large as the scientific advancements themselves. Questions arise about how extended lifespans will affect family dynamics, societal roles, and the economy. As seen in, the applications of deep generative reinforcement learning in healthcare may enhance our understanding of human biology, allowing for more personalized approaches to aging. Yet, we must also factor in behaviors and lifestyle choices that influence health. Without a comprehensive strategy addressing both technological innovation and societal adaptation, readiness for this extended life may remain an elusive goal, underscoring the need for interdisciplinary collaboration across sciences and humanities. The anticipated changes in our approach to health and wellness extend beyond mere survival; they delve into quality of life. As highlighted in, various diets and lifestyle modifications demonstrate how nutrition can serve as a significant mitigating factor in aging, yet these approaches must be promoted alongside technological enhancement. Diets such as the Mediterranean or ketogenic can foster better health outcomes and potentially extend longevity. Across various cultures, acceptance and adherence to these dietary practices will vary, presenting a considerable challenge. The societal shift towards holistic wellness necessitates informed choices from individuals, families, and communities, making education and outreach essential components of this transition. The readiness for extended life hinges not solely on scientific advancements but also on cultural readiness and the willingness to adapt to new health paradigms. Addressing the readiness for a life extended to 150 years involves grappling with the implications at both individual and collective levels. While biotechnology may offer technical solutions, societal acceptance and adaptation require a more nuanced approach. As shown in, understanding complex biological mechanisms associated with aging helps inform strategies for intervention and health management. Prolonged longevity could lead to an increased burden on healthcare systems, necessitating a robust framework for sustainable health care and resource allocation. We must reflect on our values and priorities as a society: Should we focus on extending life at all costs, or should we prioritize the quality of those additional years? Balancing these considerations will not only inform policy and research but will also be critical in ensuring that society is genuinely ready for the monumental transition toward an extended human lifespan.

REFERENCES

Division on Earth and Life Studies. 'Preparing for Future Products of Biotechnology.' National Academies of Sciences, Engineering, and Medicine, National Academies Press, 7/28/2017

United Nations. Department of Economic and Social Affairs. 'Development in an Ageing World.' UN, 1/1/2007

Colin F. Macdonald. 'Processions: Studies of Bronze Age Ritual and Ceremony presented to Robert B. Koehl.' Judith Weingarten, Archaeopress Publishing Ltd, 10/5/2023

Francesco Caputo. 'Understanding Cognitive Differences Across Cultures: Integrating Neuroscience and Cultural Psychology.' Tachia Chin, Frontiers Media SA, 11/10/2022

ChatGPT. 'The Psychology of Aging.' Understanding the Unique Perspectives and Needs of the Elderly Population, Barrett Williams, Barrett Williams, 11/22/2024

United States. Internal Revenue Service. 'Cumulative List of Organizations Described in Section 170 (c) of the Internal Revenue Code of 1954.' Department of the Treasury, Internal Revenue Service, 1/1/1990

Marvin B Sussman. 'Families.' Intergenerational and Generational Connections, Susan K Pfeifer, Routledge, 6/17/2014

Andrew J. Cherlin. 'Labor's Love Lost.' The Rise and Fall of the Working-Class Family in America, Russell Sage Foundation, 12/4/2014

Suzanne Kunkel. 'Aging, Society, and the Life Course, Fourth Edition.' Leslie A. Morgan, Springer Publishing Company, 3/15/2011

Paul Kalanithi. 'When Breath Becomes Air (Indonesian Edition).' Bentang Pustaka, 10/6/2016

William B. Schwartz. 'Coping with Methuselah.' The Impact of Molecular Biology on Medicine and Society, Henry Aaron, Rowman & Littlefield, 1/20/2004

Gilbert Meilaender. 'Should We Live Forever?.' The Ethical Ambiguities of Aging, Wm. B. Eerdmans Publishing, 1/14/2013

William B. Johnston. 'Workforce 2000.' Work and Workers for the 21st Century, Hudson Institute, 1/1/1987

Health and Medicine Division. 'Crossing the Global Quality Chasm.' Improving Health Care Worldwide, National Academies of Sciences, Engineering, and Medicine, National Academies Press, 1/27/2019

Joseph F. Coughlin. 'The Longevity Economy.' Unlocking the World's Fastest-Growing, Most Misunderstood Market, PublicAffairs, 11/7/2017

Marta Zaraska. 'Growing Young.' How Friendship, Optimism, and Kindness Can Help You Live to 100, Appetite by Random House, 6/16/2020

Health and Medicine Division. 'Preventing Cognitive Decline and Dementia.' A Way Forward, National Academies of Sciences, Engineering, and Medicine, National Academies Press, 10/5/2017

Amit Etkin. 'Handbook of Mental Health and Aging.' Nathan Hantke, Academic Press, 4/11/2020

Division of Behavioral and Social Sciences and Education. 'Social Isolation and Loneliness in Older Adults.' Opportunities for the Health Care System, National Academies of Sciences, Engineering, and Medicine, National Academies Press, 5/14/2020

Arline McDonald. 'Vitamins and Minerals.' Supplements for Wellness and Longevity, Susan Male Smith, Publications International, Limited, 1/1/2020

E.J. Masoro. 'Caloric Restriction: A Key to Understanding and Modulating Aging.' Elsevier, 12/20/2002

Gurcharan Kaur. 'Nutrition, Food and Diet in Ageing and Longevity.' Suresh I. S. Rattan, Springer Nature, 10/3/2021

Dr. M. Qassim. 'The Science of Healing Foods: Clinical Nutrition for Chronic Disease Management.' Nutritional Interventions for Diabetes, Heart Disease, Cancer, and More, Dr. M. Qassim, 9/23/2024

Hassan Chamsi-Pasha. 'Contemporary Bioethics.' Islamic Perspective, Mohammed Ali Al-Bar, Springer, 5/27/2015

National Academy of Medicine. 'Human Genome Editing.' Science, Ethics, and Governance, National Academies of Sciences, Engineering, and Medicine, National Academies Press, 8/13/2017

Sang Jin Lee. 'Organ Tissue Engineering.' Daniel Eberli, Springer International Publishing, 4/22/2021

Board on Neuroscience and Behavioral Health. 'Stem Cells and the Future of Regenerative Medicine.' Institute of Medicine, National Academies Press, 1/25/2002

Robert Lanza. 'Principles of Regenerative Medicine.' Anthony Atala, Academic Press, 12/16/2010

David Ahern. 'Oncology Informatics.' Using Health Information Technology to Improve Processes and Outcomes in Cancer, Bradford W. Hesse, Academic Press, 3/17/2016

OECD. 'Artificial Intelligence in Society.' OECD Publishing, 6/11/2019

Mamta Baunthiyal. 'Advances in Biotechnology.' Indu Ravi, Springer Science & Business Media, 10/21/2013

Klaus Schwab. 'The Fourth Industrial Revolution.' Crown, 1/3/2017

Matthew D. LaPlante. 'Lifespan.' Why We Age—and Why We Don't Have To, David A. Sinclair, Simon and Schuster, 9/10/2019

Vern L. Bengtson, PhD. 'Handbook of Theories of Aging, Second Edition.' Merril Silverstein, PhD, Springer Publishing Company, 10/27/2008

Inhee Mook-Jung. 'Aging Mechanisms.' Longevity, Metabolism, and Brain Aging, Nozomu Mori, Springer, 11/26/2015

Iris Chi. 'Successful Aging.' Asian Perspectives, Sheung-Tak Cheng, Springer, 1/26/2015

Robert L. Kahn. 'Successful Aging.' John Wallis Rowe, Random House Large Print, 1/1/1998

James C. Riley. 'Rising Life Expectancy.' A Global History, Cambridge University Press, 6/4/2001

Paola S. Timiras. 'Physiological Basis of Aging and Geriatrics.' CRC Press, 8/16/2007

Ahmed Arfa. 'Sphri exam practice questions.' 970 Challenging Questions To Prepare For SPHRI Exam, Ahmed Arfa, 9/5/2020

Division of Behavioral and Social Sciences and Education. 'Explaining Divergent Levels of Longevity in High-Income Countries.' National Research Council, National Academies Press, 6/27/2011

www.ingramcontent.com/pod-product-compliance
Lightning Source LLC
Chambersburg PA
CBHW071528220526
45469CB00003B/686